# MAGNESIUM
## Everyday Secrets

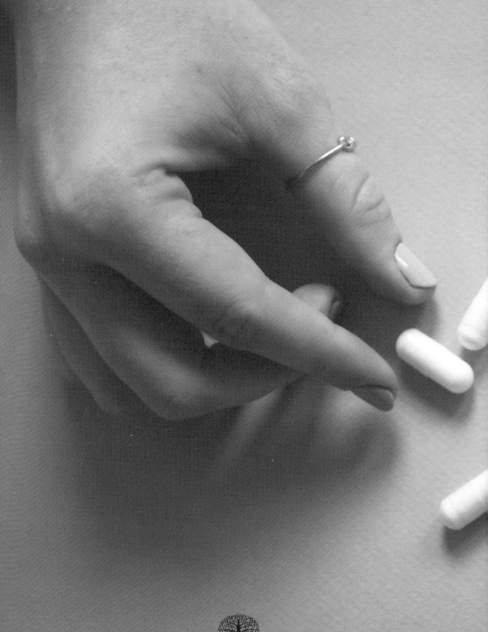

THE COUNTRYMAN PRESS
A division of W. W. Norton & Company
*Independent Publishers Since 1923*

A LIFESTYLE GUIDE TO EPSOM SALTS, MAGNESIUM OIL, AND NATURE'S RELAXATION MINERAL

# MAGNESIUM

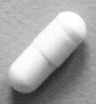

GRETCHEN LIDICKER

Additional photography by Lucia Mangione

DISCLAIMER: This volume is intended as a general information resource. It is not a substitute for, and should not be deemed to include, legal or medical advice. Dietary supplements can have or cause significant physical effects. Magnesium supplements should not be used by individuals with high or low blood pressure, or any form of heart or kidney disease, except under supervision of a medical doctor. If you have been diagnosed with, or suspect you may have, any medical or psychological condition, or if you are pregnant or considering pregnancy, consult your doctor or other professional health care provider before taking any supplement. Do not give any supplement to children or the elderly except on the advice of a doctor.

References in this book to third-party organizations, tools, products, and services are for general information purposes only. Neither the publisher nor the author can guarantee that any particular practice or resource will be useful or appropriate to the reader. Web addresses included in this book reflect links existing as of the date of first publication. The publisher is not responsible for the content of any website, blog, or information page other than its own.

For information about permission to reproduce selections from this book, write to Permissions, The Countryman Press, 500 Fifth Avenue, New York, NY 10110

For information about special discounts for bulk purchases, please contact W. W. Norton Special Sales at specialsales@wwnorton.com or 800-233-4830

Manufacturing by Versa Press
Book design by Tiani Kennedy
Production manager: Devon Zahn

The Countryman Press
www.countrymanpress.com

A division of W. W. Norton & Company, Inc.
500 Fifth Avenue, New York, NY 10110
www.wwnorton.com

978-1-68268-348-4 (pbk.)

10  9  8  7  6  5  4  3  2  1

To my friends (you know who you are),
thank you for making my heart lighter and
my days a whole lot more fun

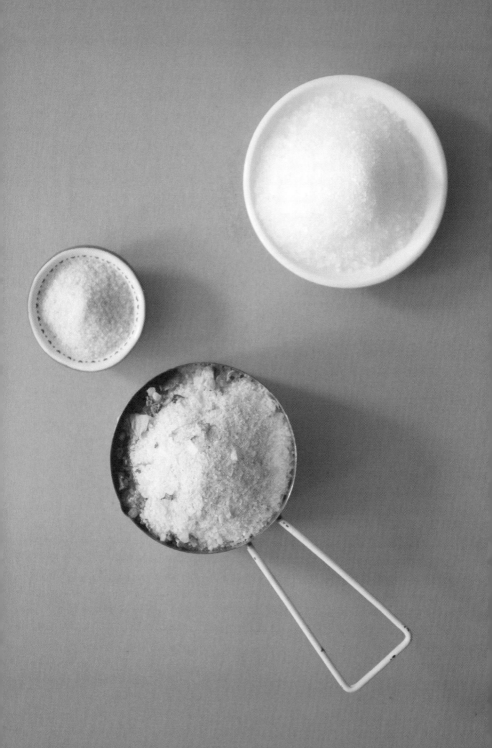

# CONTENTS

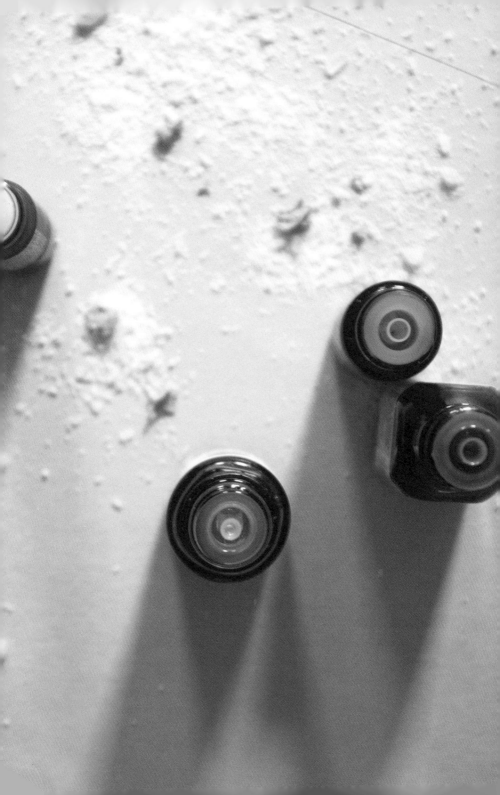

# INTRODUCTION

## Meet Magnesium, Nature's Relaxation Mineral

You've probably heard about magnesium, one of the many minerals found on earth and in the human body. Maybe your mom had you take Epsom salt baths when you were sick as a kid, or maybe you've heard that in pill form it helped a friend who suffered from chronic migraines. If you're particularly health savvy, maybe you know that some foods are higher in magnesium than others (spinach, anyone?) or that it's an important mineral for preventing and healing muscle spasms, constipation, insomnia, anxiety, blood pressure . . . I think you're catching my drift. Whatever the reason, magnesium is everywhere—in our self-care routines, our supplements, and our meals and snacks.

If you have done some research on magnesium, you likely found that supplementing your diet with it isn't as simple as you thought. Questions like "How do I know if I'm deficient?" "How much is too much?" and "What form should I take?" all need to be answered. And even if you did decide to supplement, you were undoubtedly confronted with making the choice between a bunch of different forms of magnesium, which gave you uncomfortable flashbacks to your high school chemistry class. *I mean, who really knows the difference between magnesium citrate and magnesium oxalate?* If you forged ahead anyway, you still had to choose a delivery method, a supplement brand to try, and a dosage to start with. There's a lot to think about and it can feel unnecessarily complicated.

If you asked your doctor about supplementing with magnesium or getting tested for a deficiency, the idea might have been dismissed. Most conventional doctors don't have real training in the world of supplements and—although this is a generalization—they often dismiss their value. This might have caused you to doubt the power of magnesium altogether, and you might have wondered if it's a waste of money. That's all understandable.

If you've asked yourself these questions about magnesium, or any supplement for that matter, you're definitely not alone. The world of supplements can be overwhelming, even for the most health-conscious among us. It can also feel like all the information about supplements and their value is conveniently written by people who want to sell them to you. (Suspicious.) To put the cherry on top, a study will come out that praises a certain supplement only to be closely trailed by another study that questions its level of effectiveness or its value altogether—and sometimes this all happens in the very same week. Is taking a magnesium supplement even worth your time and effort?

As the health editor at mindbodygreen, a major health and wellness media company, I navigate these choppy waters on a daily basis. In this book, you'll learn the basics of magnesium—one of the most popular supplements out there—how it works in the body, why many of us might want to take it, and how it can be a powerful tool when facing chronic stress. This book will also inform you of the many, many (many) health conditions related to a deficiency in this important mineral. And you'll learn to navigate the depths of the supplement aisle at your local health food store or on the Internet—a skill that I have acquired through years of working in integrative and functional medicine, learning from top doctors, writing and researching, and of course, through a lot—*and I mean, a lot*—of personal trial and error. You'll also notice that I recommend a few specific products, so I think it's worth noting that I have no financial connections to any of the brands I mention in the book. They're simply brands that I think are doing a nice job and that I might use myself.

The truth is, I wrote this book because I'm just as interested in how to use magnesium as a tool for better health as you are. I've worked with top doctors in the integrative and functional medicine space—including Dr. David Perlmutter, Dr. Mark Hyman, Dr. Aviva Romm, and Dr. Frank Lipman—and I'm fascinated that they all agree that magnesium is a powerful tool for better health. Even many conventional doctors are starting to suggest it to their patients. There's no doubt that magnesium is making waves.

In the last few chapters of this book, we'll have some fun with this mineral. We'll incorporate magnesium into our morning rituals, food and drinks, self-care practices, and most important, we'll bring it into our bathtubs. If you're serious about prioritizing stress management—a true act of defiance in a world that gets more hectic by the day—and want to feel better physically and mentally, this book is for you.

Are you ready? Let's get started.

# The Science of Magnesium

By now you know that magnesium is a mineral found on the planet and also inside the human body. But what does that mean, exactly? Sometimes it's hard to reconcile the idea of the magnesium on the periodic table, the white magnesium powder in a supplement capsule, and the magnesium found naturally in our bodies. Well, I'm here to tell you that it *is pretty confusing*. Magnesium is everywhere! So let's zoom out and take a big-picture look at the science of magnesium and all the different roles it plays in our body and on earth.

Magnesium is one of the most common elements found on the planet. Most of the magnesium on earth is tied up in mineral deposits, which are just naturally occurring accumulations of metals or minerals. We can't easily access these deposits of magnesium, but luckily magnesium is also plentiful in our oceans and rivers where it's generally found in its ionized form, also known as $Mg^{2+}$. We'll learn more about minerals found in water when we talk about the history of magnesium and spiritual bathing.

Magnesium plays an important role on the earth and in the lives of plants and animals, including humans. When it comes to us humans, magnesium is an essential mineral—a *mineral* is a naturally occurring chemical and the word *essential* tells us that we have to get it from food or drink because our body can't make it itself. Other essential minerals include calcium, phosphorus, potassium, sulfur, sodium, chloride, iron, zinc, copper, manganese, iodine, selenium, molybdenum, chromium, and fluoride. In nutrition, we talk a lot about vitamins and minerals, especially in the context of what can go wrong when we don't get

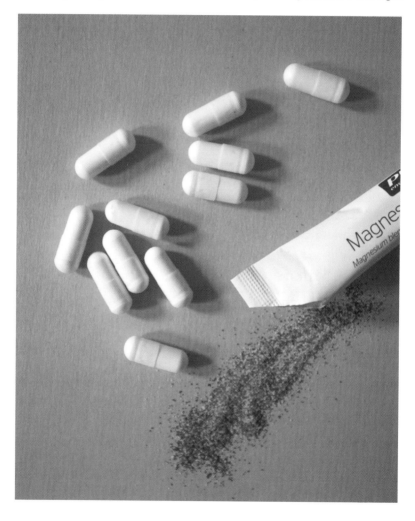

enough of them. But despite how much they're mentioned, it's easy to go through life not knowing exactly what they are.

## THE BASICS OF MAGNESIUM, VITAMINS, AND MINERALS

To put it as simply as possible, vitamins and minerals are micronutrients. As the term denotes, the body needs small amounts of them to function (as opposed to macronutrients such as protein and carbohydrates, which the body needs large amounts of). Minerals differ from vitamins because minerals are *inorganic* elements that are essential for key bodily processes, like those that help build strong bones, allow muscles to contract and relax, and keep the brain functioning as it should. I don't want to get too science-y, but when something is inorganic it means that it does not contain carbon-to-hydrogen bonds. In comparison, vitamins are *organic* compounds and essential to the body itself.

In general, minerals are more stable than vitamins, which means you don't have to worry as much about how you store them. That being said, you can lose minerals such as magnesium when you process foods. Indeed, the amount of processed foods currently in our diet puts us at risk for mineral deficiencies, including a magnesium deficiency. In addition, when grains, sugars, and oils are refined, that process removes most (or all) of the magnesium. This is a major reason why our diets are so lacking in this important mineral (more on this later in the chapter on magnesium deficiency, I promise). You can also lose minerals in other ways. For example, diets high in sodium might lead to a calcium deficiency, because when the body gets rid of excess sodium in the urine it can take calcium with it.

All vitamins and minerals are important to our health to varying degrees, and deficiencies in them can cause a wide range of side effects. $B_{12}$ deficiency, for example, can cause fatigue, poor balance, and tingling feet; and a deficiency in zinc has been associated with skin problems and immune-system dysfunction. Magnesium, in particular, has become a mineral of interest because of the wide range of symptoms and disorders associated with its deficiency in the body. These deficiencies are "widespread" and "multifaceted," according to an article published in the journal *Medical Hypotheses*.

When we talk about the role magnesium plays in our health, the best place to start is to identify where it actually exists in the body. About half of the magnesium in our body is found in our bones, and the rest is in tissues such as our muscles, nerves, and fascia. The balance of magnesium in our bodies is controlled by our kidneys. If your body needs to get rid of excess magnesium—which happens when there is more in your body than it actually needs to absorb at the time—it does so by excreting it through the urine. Interestingly, this excretion aligns itself with your circadian rhythm, also known as your "biological clock," meaning that you get rid of most of your extra magnesium at night. All the cells in your body handle magnesium differently, so a cell in your brain will have different needs than one in your liver, for example. There are over 3,700 magnesium binding sites in your body.

Knowing this, you start to understand why everyone in health and wellness is crazy about magnesium. It also won't come as a shock to learn that according to the National Institutes of Health, "Magnesium is a cofactor in more than 300 enzyme systems that regulate diverse biochemical reactions in the body." They definitely weren't exaggerating when they wrote "diverse." These biochemical reactions are involved in bodily functions that range from protein synthesis, blood sugar control, blood pressure regulation, energy production, and glycolysis to oxidative phosphorylation, bone formation, DNA synthesis, antioxidant synthesis, and calcium and potassium transport across cell membranes, just to give you some examples. If you have no idea what any of that means, don't worry. But rest assured that they are all hugely important to our health—allowing our muscles to contract, our nerves to conduct impulses, and our heart to maintain its normal healthy rhythm.

As you can imagine, this means that a deficiency in magnesium can affect our health in myriad ways. We will learn more about these effects when we cover the health benefits of magnesium in Chapter 5. For now, a few basic actions of magnesium are important to know about. The first explains why we often see magnesium paired up with another important mineral: calcium.

## THE RELATIONSHIP BETWEEN CALCIUM AND MAGNESIUM

When I say the word *calcium*, what's the first thing that comes to your mind? I'd bet big money that your answer is something like "bone health" or "build strong bones." I know for me personally, a big chunk of what I learned about nutrition during childhood had everything to

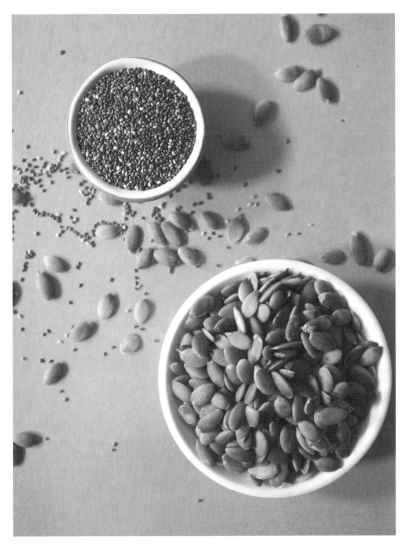

do with calcium. *Drink your milk,* they said. *It's good for your bones,* they said. Well, besides my personal issue with this advice (in the form of my longstanding intolerance to dairy), the notion that calcium and milk are the end all be all for healthy bones is misleading in a few ways.

Here's why:

For starters, the idea that dairy or calcium supplements are the best way (or the only way) to get your daily dose of calcium is just false. People are starting to take a closer look at dairy and are realizing that it isn't much of a health food at all. The dairy industry itself is another matter, where the inhumanely treated and antibiotic-laden cows pose ethical dilemmas. Dr. Tiffany Lester, an integrative medicine physician at Parsley Health—one of the leading integrative and functional medicine practices in the nation—wrote that "Milk often doesn't do a body good.... Not only does it contain IGF-1, which increases growth hormones leading to inflammation and insulin spikes, it contains less calcium than a bowl of spinach . . ." In other words, our excessive intake of milk and dairy products might be contributing to the global epidemics of chronic inflammation and type 2 diabetes. Luckily, there are a ton of delicious foods that are both healthy and high in calcium, including:

- Sea vegetables such as kelp and wakame
- Nuts and seeds
- Bone broth
- Beans and legumes
- Leafy greens
- Sardines and salmon
- Garlic
- Figs and oranges
- Soy-based products such as edamame and tofu
- Spices and herbs such as oregano, basil, and cumin

It's important to know that increasing your intake of calcium through supplementation still might not positively influence bone health. Multiple studies, including one published in the *British Medical Journal* in 2015 titled *Calcium Intake and Risk of Fracture: Systematic Review*, have shown that calcium supplements had no significant impact on bone health. In fact, a study published in the *Journal of the American Heart Association* showed that they might *increase* a person's risk of cardiovascular disease (CVD) events. Although calcium is an essential nutrient that plays an undoubtedly important role in the body and our health, the benefits of calcium supplements and calcium-rich foods (I'm looking at you, Got Milk? commercials from the '90s) have been overplayed to the point that it's not just misleading—it's dangerous.

Last, and here's where I finally tie this back to magnesium, research has shown that taking high amounts of calcium can leave you deficient in other minerals, including—you guessed it!—magnesium. These two important minerals compete with each other in the body, or as one study published in the *British Medical Journal* described it, they "antagonise each other in (re)absorption, inflammation, and many other physiological activities." The tricky thing is that having too little calcium can also interfere with your magnesium status in a negative way. It seems to be all about finding the right balance between the two.

How do we find the right balance between calcium and magnesium for bone health, nervous system health, and overall health? For people without a serious deficiency in either nutrient, many experts recommend taking calcium and magnesium together—and eating calcium- and magnesium-rich foods together as well. But how much of each do you need? I'm glad you asked because that's what I'm about to tackle next.

## UNDERSTANDING CALCIUM-TO-MAGNESIUM RATIOS

If you're paying a visit to your friendly neighborhood health food store and you're looking at calcium-magnesium combo supplements, you'll find a lot of different ratios of calcium to magnesium. So how do you choose? The "perfect" ratio of calcium to magnesium for humans is hard to pin down, but the best ratio for you depends on your specific needs and how balanced your intake of calcium- and magnesium-rich foods is.

I'll start with the daily intake recommendations for each. The recommendations for calcium intake are all over the map. They are especially high in the United States, where adults are instructed to take more than 1,000 milligrams per day. Meanwhile, the World Health Organization (WHO) says less than 500 milligrams of calcium per day is optimal. Magnesium intake recommendations typically fall between 300 and 450 milligrams per day depending on your gender. Historically, many experts have recommended taking a 2:1 ratio of calcium to magnesium, but a growing number are starting to recommend a 1:1 ratio or even a reverse 2:1 ratio, meaning the supplement would contain twice as much magnesium as calcium. There are a few reasons for this recommendation, but the primary reason is because most people are getting enough (if not too much) calcium through supplements and their diet. This has contributed to widespread deficiencies in magnesium, so the ratios are being adjusted to restore balance, which means giving us a little more magnesium and pulling back on calcium just a bit.

When it comes to eating calcium- and magnesium-rich foods, they are best eaten together in similar quantities. You don't want to eat a ton of calcium-rich foods without magnesium there to maintain a balance between the two—or vice versa. Remember, everything in the body is connected. In fact, there's reason to believe that your body's magnesium levels and ability to absorb magnesium are affected by your vitamin $B_6$, vitamin D, potassium, and vitamin $K_2$ status on top of your calcium status.

Before I move on, there's something important to note here. When it comes to supplements—and vitamins and minerals especially—it's easy to get lost in the nitty-gritty details of what is paired best with what, what to take when, and whether taking one nutrient is useless without taking the other. These are all great considerations, and sometimes the best way to pair supplements to make them more effective is pretty clear. Vitamin D and $K_2$, for example, should always be paired together. Adding black pepper to turmeric increases its bioavailability exponentially—you'll rarely ever see one without the other. Other times, however, we're still not sure exactly what the right answer is, and trying to pair every single nutrient with its counterparts can make your head spin.

This dilemma is another reason why a food-first approach to health is always best. When you eat a wide range of fruits, veggies, healthy fats, and whole grains you're getting a wide range of different nutrients at the same time (instead of with a supplement, which might provide one or a few at a time), and many of them work synergistically. Isn't nature amazing? You'll also notice that many of the calcium-rich foods I listed previously are also on the list of magnesium-rich foods. Eating real foods will help you cover your bases and reduce the chance that you'll be severely deficient in any specific nutrient, or that you'll take too much of one nutrient that tends to crowd out another (*cough, cough:*

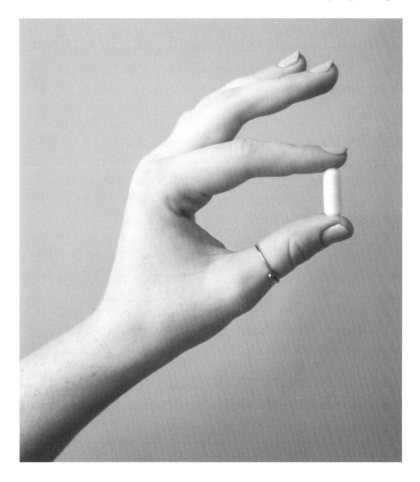

*calcium*). It's important not to forget that supplements are meant to do exactly that: supplement a healthy diet and cover any weak spots you might have from deficiencies or complicating factors.

## A WORD ON MAGNESIUM AND ELECTROLYTES

Magnesium is also often referred to as an electrolyte, which is a word that gets thrown around a lot in the health and fitness industries, but many of us aren't entirely clear on what it means. It's actually a somewhat confusing concept: A scientist would define the word differently than, say, a high school soccer coach (toss me a lemon-lime Gatorade, won't you?).

So what is an electrolyte? In the science world, magnesium, calcium, potassium, phosphate, and sodium are all considered electrolytes because they are compounds that produce ions when dissolved in water. Pretty simple. These ions can be positive or negative (magnesium is positive and chlorine is negative, for example). In the world of nutrition, fitness, and hydration we talk about electrolytes in terms of minerals that dissolve in the *body's* fluids.

More specifically, electrolytes such as sodium and potassium work together to maintain fluid balance inside and outside cells (as a result cells don't shrivel up or expand too much, a very important job). When you're eating a healthy diet, you get a lot of your electrolytes from foods. But if you sweat a lot, you tend to lose massive amounts of electrolytes and you might need to replenish your levels with more than you can typically get in your normal, everyday diet. If you live or work in a hot environment, for example, you'll need more fluids and a higher electrolyte intake. In every liter of sweat, you lose 900 mg of sodium, 15 mg of potassium, and 13 mg of magnesium.

And now the question you've all been waiting for: Should you be drinking electrolyte sports drinks? In their defense, most sports drinks do contain electrolytes to replenish your body after a workout, but they also often contain a ton of added sugar and artificial colors and flavors that aren't doing your body any favors. A regular 32-ounce bottle of Gatorade contains more than 50 grams of sugar, and while that's slightly less than a soda, researchers still think sports drinks are contributing to the epidemic of childhood obesity and tooth decay. Plus, if you're consuming these drinks on days that you are not active, you're really just adding unnecessary sodium to your diet that you likely don't need.

When you think about electrolytes, coconut water might also come to mind. Coconut water has quickly become the Gatorade of the 2010s. While it is a great source of potassium, it's actually very low in sodium, which is the most important electrolyte to replenish because, as we just learned, you lose *a lot* of salt when you sweat. So does the perfect recovery drink exist? It does! And it's conveniently described on page 110 of this book. For all you athletes out there, I created a recovery drink that's full of the important electrolytes you lose during a particularly sweaty workout—*sans* the sugar, artificial flavors, and highlighter-like colors.

And so, those are the basics of how magnesium works in the body. You now know why it's important to understand magnesium's relationship with calcium and exactly what people mean when they refer to magnesium as an electrolyte. The more you learn about this mineral and its role in the many happenings going on in your body, the more important you realize it is. But bone health and workout recovery are far from where the benefits of magnesium end. By far, magnesium is most famous for its ability to induce relaxation and to ease muscle tension. This brings us to the next chapter, which is all about learning how to relax for the sake of your health, why you're so stressed out in the first place, and how magnesium can help with both.

# 2

# The Epidemic of Chronic Stress—and How Magnesium Can Help

Let me ask you a question: Are you stressed out? I'd be surprised if you answered that question with anything other than a simple and resounding "Yes." It always amazes me that in a world full of people living totally different lives—with different stories, opinions, careers, and geographical locations—we can all agree on a few things and one of them is that stress is real, it's pervasive, and most of us are suffering from it and its unwelcome side effects.

A lot of the time it's actually easier to pinpoint moments throughout the day when we aren't stressed than those when we are. We're rushing to get out of the house in the morning and we're stressed at work. It feels like every day is just a little shorter than the day before, and yet we have more responsibilities now than we did just 24 hours ago. We're anxious about politics, about money, about the future of the planet, and about our living situation and our careers. We're stressed about our community, our friendships, aging, and our health. In an article published in the *Yale Journal of Biology and Medicine*, Margaret Reynolds wrote: "We lament about being stressed, brag about being stressed, attempt to fix and treat our stress, and (in some perverse effort to cover all our bases) stress that we are too stressed out." I don't know about you, but for me that really hits home.

We could easily compare stress to a big ugly monster stomping through our streets, tearing buildings apart and plucking cars from the roads. But actually, it's much scarier than that. Stress is more of a silent epidemic, something that's affecting us all but we feel we should be able to handle it. We are more anxious, frazzled, and stimulated than ever before. At the same time, unhealthy levels of stress are becoming more and more normal; it's a dangerous cycle and it doesn't seem to be letting up anytime soon.

## THE MENTAL, PHYSICAL, AND EMOTIONAL CONSEQUENCES OF CHRONIC STRESS

So what are the consequences of constant anxiety and stimulation of our nervous systems? I don't want to stress you out (yes, I too see the irony here) but the consequences are pretty dire. Stress seems to play a role in almost every illness out there. The American Psychological Association reports that chronic stress is directly linked to the six leading causes of death—heart disease, cancer, lung ailments, accidents, cirrhosis of the liver, and suicide—and more than 75 percent of doctor visits are for stress-related ailments and complaints.

On the list of reasons for these visits to the doctor are headaches, asthma, depression and anxiety, chronic muscle tension, poor thyroid function, weight gain, indigestion, arthritis, blood sugar imbalance, decreased bone density and muscle tissue, nausea, yeast and urinary tract infections, and even colds and sinus infections. And yes, all of these are stress-related ailments. Chronically triggering your fight-or-flight response affects your ability to stay healthy and also your ability to heal. It's nothing to mess around with, and we'd all be doing ourselves a big favor if we were able to make a dent in the amount of stress our bodies and minds take on each day.

## THE INS AND OUTS OF HOW OUR BODIES RESPOND TO STRESSFUL SITUATIONS

Our bodies were intricately designed to deal with short-term anxiety-inducing situations, such as being chased by a dog or surviving a tornado. In fact, when we're confronted with a stressor, our body does some pretty amazing things to help us. The specific order of operations our bodies follow in response to stress is really intricate, but I think it's worth explaining the basics because it's really that impressive. It all begins with our sympathetic nervous system (SNS), which is also known as the fight-or-flight part of the nervous system. Basically, when we confront a stressor the SNS sends signals to our adrenal glands that sit on top of our kidneys. The adrenals respond by releasing adrenaline into our bloodstream and that adrenaline begins to circulate throughout the body.

As a result of the release of these signals and hormones, our heart rate increases, our breathing becomes shallow, glucose is released into our bloodstream, our muscles tense, our blood vessels and airways constrict or dilate, and we actually slow down digestion so that we can direct that blood flow to other areas of the body. (If you've ever tried to eat when you were stressed and got a stomachache, became bloated, or experienced acid reflux, you've seen this gut-nervous system connection in action.)

This response is like a built-in priority system for our survival, which is pretty amazing—especially when you realize that this all happens before you really consciously become aware of what's going on. The brain also activates the HPA axis, which consists of the hypothalamus, the pituitary gland, and the adrenal glands. This keeps your body in fight-or-flight mode by setting off a hormone cascade that eventually causes the adrenals to release cortisol, which is also known as our primary "stress" hormone.

## AN INTRODUCTION TO THE PARASYMPATHETIC NERVOUS SYSTEM AND THE VAGUS NERVE

When whatever triggered our stress response passes and the threat is over, our parasympathetic nervous system (PNS) is supposed to kick in. The PNS is known as the rest and digest system, and it acts like a brake pedal that calms the nervous system when the ordeal is over and brings us back to relaxation, allowing the body to focus on other things such as digesting whatever is in the stomach.

One of the most fascinating parts of our human physiology is how we go about exercising the powers of the PNS, which all happens by way of something called the vagus nerve. This prolific nerve runs from the base of the brain through the neck and then branches out into the chest, stretching all the way down to the abdomen. The word *vagus* means "wandering" in Latin—and that's exactly what the vagus nerve does; it wanders down the body, touching the heart and almost all major organs along the way. This nerve has long been thought of as a remarkable internal sensory system because it works to regulate breathing, heart rate, muscles, digestion, circulation, and even the vocal cords.

If you haven't heard of the vagus nerve, you're not alone. And it might be because, although scientists know it has many functions, they aren't sure *exactly* how this nerve actually works. What we do know is that it's a major regulator of the peripheral nervous system because of its ability to slow the pulse and lower blood pressure. The vagus nerve is also a central player in the gut-brain axis, which is becoming more important every day as we learn more about the intricate connection between gut health and brain health. (If you've ever lost your appetite when you're nervous, you've seen this connection in action.)

Despite the fact that the PNS and the vagus nerve are looking out for us after a stressful event, a lot of the time they don't get the chance to bring our bodies back to a state of calm. This is because for the PNS to be activated, the SNS has to actually turn off. Unfortunately, our bodies and brains aren't that great at distinguishing between encountering a bear in the woods and getting stuck in traffic and receiving a rude email from a colleague. This means that all day we are continuously triggering our sympathetic nervous system, which stimulates our adrenals and HPA axis, causing the whole system to be totally overworked. It's this chronic overstimulation that contributes to the stress-related health issues that plague so many of us and prevents the PNS from being able to do what it does best.

## UNDERSTANDING MAGNESIUM'S ROLE IN THE NERVOUS SYSTEM

You might be wondering why I'm going through all this with you, especially in such detail. *This is a book about magnesium, not chronic stress, right?* Well, it turns out that magnesium plays a pivotal role in the health and activity of the parasympathetic nervous system. In fact, magnesium plays a crucial role in the nervous system in general, with studies showing that a deficiency in magnesium can induce unwanted sympathetic excitation. Basically, not having enough magnesium can trigger your flight-or-flight response and prevent your PNS from taking the reins.

Magnesium might be able to help your body cope with chronic stress and lessen the negative side effects of it. Authors of a study published in a German journal called *Fortschritte der Medizin* in 2016

### Positive Stress

Is there such a thing as healthy stress? Actually, yes. Putting your body and brain through certain amounts of stress can be great for you. In fact, it might be one of the healthiest things you can do for yourself. Dr. Dean Sherzai and Dr. Ayesha Sherzai—physicians and authors of the bestselling book *The Alzheimer's Solution*—are experts in all things brain health, but especially those that relate to lifestyle change. They talk and write a lot about the need for positive stress, which includes things such as studying hard to earn a degree that will make life easier in the future or challenging yourself to pick up a new hobby that puts you way outside your comfort zone. In an article for mindbodygreen they wrote, "Positive stress sends your neural-endocrine axis on an entirely different journey than negative stress—one that strengthens brain health by creating additional neuro-connections and reducing inflammation. Positive stress can actually be the strongest link in the chain to protecting your long-term brain health." The take-home here? Avoiding stress altogether isn't the key to health—and we need to stop lumping all stress into one big category. It's all about identifying the different types of stress in your life, categorizing it, prioritizing, and generally increasing the positive kind of stress while decreasing the negative kind.

concluded that "The results of this study point out that persons with mental and physical stress can benefit from a daily intake of magnesium. This might lead to an improved physiological regulation of the sympathetic and parasympathetic efferents and, furthermore, prevent magnesium deficiency and diseases such as, for example, restlessness, irritability, lack of concentration, sleep disorder or depression." To tie magnesium further to chronic stress, it's also thought that chronic stress depletes our body's magnesium levels. As you can imagine, this creates a vicious cycle of too much stress, too little magnesium, more stress, less magnesium . . . I think you can see how this could quickly spin out of control.

The impact of stress on our health is something that both conventional doctors and integrative and functional medicine doctors can agree on. That said, in more holistic circles they talk a lot about something called "adrenal fatigue" as well, which is a condition that is not yet accepted in conventional spaces. Essentially, adrenal fatigue is a mild form of adrenal insufficiency that occurs when your adrenal glands (which are responsible for producing the hormones adrenaline and cortisol) are so overworked that they stop functioning like they should. According to Dr. Aviva Romm—a leading integrative medicine doctor, herbalist, midwife, and author of the book *The Adrenal Thyroid Revolution*—some common symptoms of adrenal fatigue are:

- Extreme fatigue and lethargy
- Sleep problems
- Irritability, anxiety, feeling blue
- Sugar, carbs, fat, caffeine, or salt cravings
- Tiredness around 3 or 4 p.m.
- Weight gain, especially around your middle
- Getting sick more often than you used to
- Hormonal problems and imbalances
- Brain fog and forgetfulness
- Digestive issues
- Hashimoto's symptoms or another autoimmune condition

Basically, you feel tired, stressed, burnt out, overwhelmed, and unable to take on the day. You'll also likely feel tired all day and then completely amped in the evenings when you're trying to fall asleep, due to a dysregulation in your circadian rhythm and cortisol-melatonin cycle.

Sadly, symptoms like these are either brushed off by doctors or misdiagnosed as something else—like anxiety or depression—especially in women. If this sounds all too familiar to you, I recommend you see a doctor who is well-versed in looking at adrenal health in a holistic way, such as an integrative medicine doctor or naturopathic doctor. Healing from adrenal fatigue requires more than just your average stress-busting techniques like meditation and yoga. More often than not, doctors will suggest a targeted supplement regime, dietary changes, for instance, cutting out caffeine and sugar, and focusing on restorative exercise and increasing sleep quality.

## HOW NOT TO GET TOO STRESSED OUT ABOUT CHRONIC STRESS

You might feel like this chapter is all about the problem without offering any solutions. But there's a lot you can do to empower yourself and punch chronic stress right in the face. So are you ready for some good news? You'll be happy to know that fighting stress doesn't necessarily require expensive supplements or technology or even a membership to a meditation or yoga studio. Effective stress-combating strategies can be anything from spending more time face-to-face with friends to avoiding technology in the evenings to getting an hour or two more of sleep each night. Meditation is another great way to train yourself to handle stress. Research has shown that mindfulness meditation actually changes the way our brains respond to stressors, which means it tempers the fight-or-flight response we just talked about and strengthens the vagus nerve, which regulates the PNS. You don't need apps or expensive classes to meditate—just sit down, close your eyes, and breathe in and out slowly through your nose 25 times. Try to make your exhales longer than your inhales, and make sure your shoulders are relaxed and that when you inhale you're breathing into your belly instead of your upper chest.

It pains me to say it but I have to deliver some not-so-good news along with the good news. The truth is that finding an enjoyable way to reduce stress isn't the hard part (there are about a million fun, cheap, easy ways to do it). The challenge is actually making time in your day *to do it*. When we're running from obligation to obligation, it's so tempting to tell ourselves that we're too busy to take a few minutes to reduce stress. Unfortunately, many of us will give ourselves that exact same line for years on end. And we already know what the consequences of that will be. It's not a matter of if stress will catch up to us, it's a matter of when and how badly it will come back to haunt us.

With this book, my goal is to inspire you to prioritize self-care and to make stress reduction a serious part of your daily routine—and to use magnesium as a secret weapon to help make it happen. It's a happy coincidence that magnesium can be used in a lot of different ways, and many of them force us to put down the phone and take a few minutes for ourselves. Win-win!

At the end of the day, we can't prevent the bus being delayed, the kids getting sick right before a big presentation at work, or the line at the grocery store that winds all the way back to the bathrooms. We also can't prevent the hardships and losses we'll all suffer at one point or another, and the grief and anxiety that come with them. We can, however, give our body some tender loving care and do what we can to mitigate the negative consequences of these stressors (big and small) on our health. And that's something worth learning about!

As Dr. Ellen Vora—an integrative psychiatrist who I've worked closely with for years—once wrote:

If you want to decrease stress, begin to shift away from phones, screens, social media, fluorescent cubicles, shopping, clutter, sterile environments, dings, pings, notifications, and addiction to busyness, and shift toward nature, stillness, slow food, dirt, bugs, physical con-

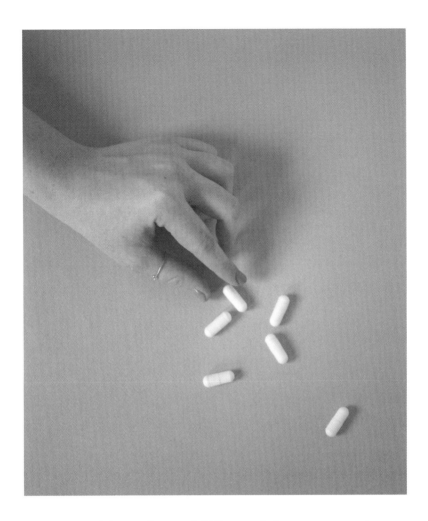

nection with human beings, fulfilling work, living more simply, owning less stuff, and doing less overall. I'm asking you to go beyond simply reading a book about minimalist home décor; I'm telling you to hurl your phone across the room and choose how you spend the moments of your life!

What are you waiting for?

# 3

# The History of Magnesium, Epsom Salts, and Spiritual Bathing

Now that we know about the science of magnesium and its potential for helping with the big problem of chronic stress, it's time to turn to the history of this natural remedy. This history includes Epsom salts and spiritual bathing. While supplementing with magnesium and other minerals in this way might feel like a modern wellness trend, its history is actually long, rich, and part of nearly every culture.

The tradition of bathing in salt water begins where you might expect: the sea. Seawater is a conveniently plentiful source of magnesium and other minerals. The ocean's average concentration of magnesium is about 55 mmol/L (millimole per liter), and the Dead Sea, which is known for being one of the richest sources of minerals on the planet, has a magnesium concentration of more than 198 mmol/L. To compare, the concentration of magnesium in human blood serum is only about 0.8 mmol/L. And it's not just magnesium; a lot of the minerals in seawater have wonderful healing properties that are worth knowing about and experimenting with.

## THE HISTORY OF HEALING BATHS AND TRANSDERMAL MAGNESIUM THERAPY

People have been bathing in seawater (and therefore, taking advantage of transdermal magnesium therapy) for thousands of years. Even as early as 2700 BC a text was published that discussed more than 40 different kinds of salt and how to use them. Hippocrates, who is well known as the father of modern medicine, suggested using seawater for healing, especially for patients with aching muscles and arthritis. The ancient Greeks soaked in seawater and heated seaweed (a rich source of magnesium) baths. What's more, drinking seawater for health was part of many ancient cultures.

In the mid-1700s, Dr. Charles Russell published a book entitled *The Uses of Sea Water,* which gave instructions on how to use mineral-rich seawater to treat various diseases. Bath products containing Dead Sea salts (which contains at least 21 minerals, including magnesium, calcium, sulfur, bromide, iodine, sodium, zinc, and potassium) were thought to provide relief from various skin diseases. They might not have been able to explain why, but many ancient cultures knew that long soaks in certain waters helped with various health woes. People didn't just bathe in the ocean, they also bathed in hot springs and lakes and rivers—some of which are great sources of magnesium.

So where do Epsom salts come in? Epsom salts were discovered in the early 17th century, in a town about 15 miles from London, called—you'll never guess—Epsom. According to various historical accounts, there was a bitter saline spring in the town and it was discovered that bathing in the water could help heal wounds more quickly, and drinking it had a laxative effect. People traveled to the town from all over Europe to take advantage of its healing properties. The town quickly turned into one of the first spa experience destinations. Eventually, people discovered that boiling the water produced magnesium sulfate salts. This process enabled the salts to be transported and sold more easily.

Epsom salts were officially named by a chemist named Nehemiah Grew, who described them in his book about "bitter purging salts." He was the first person to sell Epsom salts and provide them to people as an over-the-counter remedy. Today, magnesium sulfate and other forms of magnesium are FDA-approved laxatives, used by both conventional and holistic practitioners. High-end resorts and spas still offer various ritual healing baths on their spa menus as ways to improve skin quality and circulation, and even to lose weight and detoxify. There are also float spas, a form of sensory deprivation chamber, where you float in extremely buoyant, mineral-rich water in total darkness.

It's pretty cool to think that even today, hundreds of years later, Epsom salts are still sold in giant bags at most major grocery stores, pharmacies, and health food stores. Of course, now magnesium oils, creams, and supplements are available in capsule, powder, and liquid form. So for those of you who thought magnesium might just be another passing wellness trend, think again!

## THE SPIRITUAL SIDE OF BATHING AND HOW TO CREATE A RITUAL OUT OF YOUR MAGNESIUM BATH

You've probably deduced this already, but there is a definitive spiritual theme weaving through the history of healing baths. Spiritual bathing has long been thought of as a way to achieve higher consciousness or wash away impurities. Water is often considered to be sacred, and it is used to cleanse and purify the spirit and wash away negative influences. In her book *Spiritual Bathing: Healing Rituals and Traditions from Around the World*, Rosita Arvigo—a traditional healer, doctor of naturopathy, herbalist, and ethnobotanist—wrote that "nearly all cultures equate water with energy. . . . Since ancient times people have firmly believed that energy carried by water can transform human energy. This is central to the understanding of the effect of spiritual bathing." Almost every culture features water or bathing somewhere in their practices and rituals: the Incas, Native Americans, Muslims, Christians, Buddhists, and the Celts and Druids.

Whether you're religious or spiritual or not, I encourage you to utilize the bath recipes in the second half of this book. At the very least, you can make an experience out of them. Breathe deeply, be mindful, turn off your phone, and take those few minutes for yourself. It doesn't

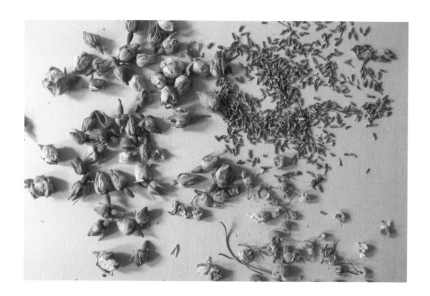

have to be a spiritual practice, but it can be a practice in mindfulness and self-care. Here are some quick guidelines to get the most out of an Epsom salt bath or any of the magnesium-inspired recipes in this book:

1. Find a time in the day (I prefer right before bed) when you won't feel rushed and can dedicate at least 30 minutes to yourself. Decide in advance which bath recipe you're going to use.

2. Clean your bathtub with a cleaner that is free from harsh chemicals. Make sure you'll feel totally comfortable and content lying down for 20 minutes or so.

3. Run the water and use this time to tidy up the bathroom and get the lighting just right—you don't want any glaring overhead lights. Maybe light a candle or two or three, go crazy!

4. Add the salts to the bath while the water is still running (this will help them dissolve), then turn off the water and add the other ingredients (essential oils, herbs, flowers, and so forth).

5. Leave your phone off and put it in another room. If you want to listen to some music using your phone, then bring it in. Just be sure to silence the ringer or put it in airplane mode so that you can stay fully present.

6. Once you're in the water, simply breathe and let your mind idle. It's the perfect moment to sort through the things on your mind, allow your subconscious thoughts to flow, and to give your feelings the space and time they need to show their faces.

7. Try to activate your senses—feel the water on your skin, notice its temperature, and gently inhale the smells of whatever ingredients you've decided to use in the bath.

8. When you leave the bath, take a few minutes to transition back to your day or evening. Be still and allow yourself to feel the effects of the magnesium on your body and mind. How do your muscles feel? How is your mood? Reflect just a little bit before you move on.

## BEYOND THE CAPSULE: HOW TO TURN MAGNESIUM SUPPLEMENTATION INTO SELF-CARE

This might all feel a little too "woo-woo" for you, and I get it. If that's the case, simply think of your bath as a self-check-in. Dr. Tieraona Low Dog, a physician and pioneer in the field of integrative medicine, once said, "A daily spiritual bath is an easy way to start paying attention to your spirit and soul as well as your body." Simple as that!

This mindful strategy can also be applied to the benefits of the recipes in this book. It would be quick and easy to just pop a few magnesium capsules each day but that would be missing the point. Incorporating magnesium into your self-care routine and creating moments and rituals around it encourages you to slow down and get in touch with your body and your needs. So don't rush it! A big factor at play in the chronic stress many of us are experiencing is the illusion that everything needs to be done as fast as humanly possible.

One last thing before I move on: I want to talk directly to those of you who are feeling guilty for taking this time for yourself or are feeling overly indulgent for drawing yourself a luxurious bubble bath. The truth is this: If you can't show up for yourself, how the heck are you going to show up for somebody else? A very smart person once said, "You can't pour from an empty cup." I'm not sure if wiser words have ever been spoken.

Luxurious baths aren't everyone's cup of tea. If you're struggling to relax because you can't quite justify this act of self-love, try repeating a mantra while you're ignoring your phone, email, to-do list, and any and all intrusive thoughts. Currently, my favorite one is: *Right now, I am not responsible for anything.* I love the idea of giving yourself permission to put it all down—even if just temporarily—and enjoying the freedom of looking out for numero uno (that would be you).

I like a modern wellness trend as much as the next person, but there's something really nice about knowing that magnesium and Epsom salt baths have stood the test of time. It gives them a certain credibility and reminds me that even without modern technology and a vast body of scientific knowledge, humans have always been creative and ingenuous.

# Magnesium Deficiencies

The world of supplements can be overwhelming. I mean, with all the thousands of options out there, where do you even begin? Even I—someone who's been smack in the middle of the health and wellness industry for years—can get overwhelmed. I can also admit that, despite my ever-growing expertise, I've wasted my fair share of money on supplements that I never ended up taking. Seemingly every new brand or product claims that it is superior to any other on the market. What I've learned over the years is this: When it comes to supplements, approach them with a critical eye, and don't get lost in all marketing and excellent packaging that makes you feel like you need to take all of them. *You do not need to take all of them.* Supplementing is all about targeting a specific problem and applying a specific dose and form of a nutrient.

## NAVIGATING THE WONDERFUL WORLD OF SUPPLEMENTS

Supplements are a lot more complicated than just self-identifying a problem, heading to the drugstore, and taking the recommended dose on the back of the bottle. If you do approach it this way, you probably won't have much success. And this is an important point: There are a lot of people out there using supplements incorrectly or buying low-quality products, taking them for a couple of weeks without making any other changes in their lifestyle, and then dismissing them as ineffective when they don't work. To add to that, many studies on supplements don't account for varying quality among brands or even the form of the nutrient used. There's a big gap between just "taking supplements" and taking supplements the way they were meant to be taken.

When working with health care practitioners, I'm often surprised when they tell me to take only half the dose or sometimes three times the dose recommended on the bottle. Other times, I've been instructed to take certain supplements only during certain times of the month, or times of day, or pair certain supplements with very specific lifestyle changes. These are things you just can't know on your own; these are the details that supplement-savvy health care practitioners have learned through years and years of clinical practice and observation.

That's why, these days, when I'm thinking about experimenting with a new supplement—and dropping the money to buy it—I make sure that (1) I actually need it and it's not just the latest trend; (2) I'm taking the right dose and form for what I'm trying to accomplish; and (3) I'm buying from a brand that goes above and beyond when it comes to quality and potency. This way, I avoid the supplement graveyard that many of us are all too familiar with. Isn't it nice to be a little older and wiser?

## HOW TO KNOW IF YOU NEED A MAGNESIUM SUPPLEMENT

So how do you know if you really need to be taking magnesium? The answer to this question isn't entirely cut-and-dry, but I'll start by telling you that the 2005–2006 National Health and Nutrition Examination Survey (NHANES) showed that at least 50 percent of American adults had inadequate intakes of magnesium, making it one of the most common deficiency in adults. This lack of magnesium is frequently referred to as the "invisible deficiency." Why is this, exactly? We already know that too much calcium puts us at risk for magnesium deficiency, but we're also not getting as much magnesium in our diet as we did in the past. We have the standard American diet (and our obsession with calcium intake) to thank for that. Magnesium and other essential nutrients are also typically lost or diminished when we harvest, process, store, refrigerate, and transport food. For example, grains used to be a decent source of magnesium, but the refined white bread many people eat today is basically devoid of the mineral altogether. The consequences of this are pretty severe. In fact, one study published in the *Open Heart* even concluded that magnesium deficiency is a principal driver of cardiovascular disease, describing it as a public health crisis. Are you paying attention yet? I thought so.

Knowing all this, the first question to ask yourself when it comes to a magnesium deficiency—and whether or not you might have one—is: How many magnesium-rich foods are you eating on a regular basis? Those foods include:

- Green leafy vegetables, such as spinach, kale, collard greens, turnip greens, and mustard greens
- Legumes such as black beans and lentils

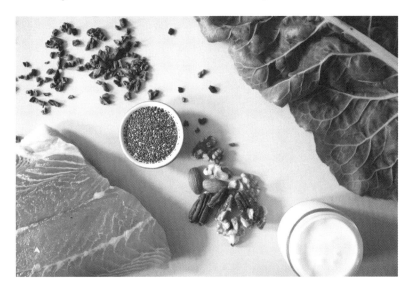

- Fruit such as figs, avocados, and bananas
- Nuts and seeds, especially pumpkin seeds, squash seeds, sesame seeds, almonds, and cashews
- Whole grains
- Yogurt and kefir
- Fatty fish such as salmon, mackerel, halibut, and tuna
- Dark chocolate

Are you eating these foods regularly and in large quantities? The recommended daily allowance for adults from the National Institutes of Health is between 310 and 320 mg of magnesium for women and 400 to 420 mg for men each day, but estimates put the average intake for adults in the United States at more like 250 milligrams daily. Where do you think you fall?

### Magnesium in Our Water Supply

We know that magnesium occurs naturally on earth and in the ocean, so you might wonder if there's magnesium in our drinking water. Well, that depends on which kind of water you're drinking. Tap, mineral, and bottled waters can range anywhere from 1 mg/L to more than 120 mg/L of magnesium, depending on where you are. Mineral-rich water is often described as "hard water." By contrast, "soft water" is water that has been treated so that the only mineral left is salt. As a general rule, you can assume that bottled and tap water won't help you get your daily dose of magnesium, although it might behoove you to check and see what the magnesium content of your water source might be so that you can know whether or not it puts you at a greater risk (or lesser risk) for deficiency. Some people believe that all of our drinking water should be infused with magnesium (like we did with fluoride in the 1940s), because of the widespread nature of its deficiency. Personally, I like to be in charge of what I'm putting in my body and when. Adding something to your water is easier than taking it out.

## FOOD ISN'T ENOUGH: ADDITIONAL FACTORS THAT PUT YOU AT RISK FOR A MAGNESIUM DEFICIENCY

If you're eating your fair share of magnesium-rich foods, is that enough to keep you safe from a deficiency? I'd be remiss if I didn't address the simple fact that our food has changed drastically in the last hundred years. Even if we're eating spinach all the time, we have to consider modern farming practices and soil quality. The fact is, there's a lower concentration of minerals in the soil today than there was even 10 years ago.

The other thing to consider is that even if you're getting adequate amounts of magnesium through your meals and snacks, you have a few other things working against you. These include, for one, the widespread use of medications—both prescription and over-the-counter—that deplete our bodies of magnesium. These medications include blood pressure meds, birth control pills, proton pump inhibitors (commonly prescribed for acid reflux and heartburn), and diuretics. In addition, digestive disorders can cause malabsorption of magnesium, which is often exacerbated by antibiotics and other prescription medications that disturb the gut microbiome. And finally, diabetes (especially if it's poorly controlled), alcohol use, caffeine intake, chronic stress, excessive sweating, heavy menstrual periods, hormone imbalances, and renal disease can all also affect your magnesium status. Magnesium deficiencies become more common with age; research shows that a person's diet tends to include less magnesium as they age, that they are more likely to take magnesium-depleting medications the older they get, and that their bodies excrete it in higher amounts as time goes by.

Like I said, knowing whether or not you're deficient in magnesium isn't exactly cut-and-dry. But I'd be surprised to find a person who didn't have at least one of these risk factors currently at play or present somewhere in their health history. At the end of the day, all of these factors can interfere with your ability to consume magnesium in the first place, as well as your ability to actually absorb and use the magnesium you're consuming. Knowing all this, I'll let you do the math on how likely it is that you're deficient.

## GETTING YOUR MAGNESIUM LEVELS TESTED: IS IT WORTH IT?

At this point you might be thinking, *why are we playing this guessing game? Can't we just get a blood test that measures our magnesium levels and then we'd know for sure if we're deficient?* It would be ideal if we could simply measure our magnesium levels with a blood test like we do for vitamins D or B$_{12}$. But sadly, finding out if you're deficient in magnesium through a test is easier said than done. And that's primarily because most of the magnesium in your body is found inside your cells and bones, which means that only about 1 percent of your body's total magnesium is circulating through your bloodstream. You can get a blood test to measure magnesium concentration, but the number you get won't tell you much about your total body magnesium levels or about the magnesium levels in specific locations in the body. This means you could have a deficiency and be experiencing symptoms (such as fatigue, cognitive issues, and headaches) but a serum magnesium concentration test could come back completely normal.

You can also measure magnesium by assessing magnesium or ionized magnesium concentrations in red blood cells, saliva, and urine. The magnesium test available appears to be the magnesium "tolerance test," which is when urine magnesium levels are measured after administering magnesium through an IV or a shot. This test works because, if you remember, magnesium homeostasis—or the amount of magnesium your body decides to keep around or get rid of—is controlled by the kidneys. Simply, when you have too much magnesium, the body releases it through your urine. On any typical day, you'll lose about 120 mg of magnesium. When your overall magnesium status is low, you'll have less than that in your urine because your body will try to hold on to it. If your urine has low levels of magnesium after the shot or IV, your health care practitioner might conclude that you're likely deficient, as your body gobbled up all the magnesium it was given. If there's a bunch of magnesium in your urine, then your health care practitioner could assume your levels were in a good place because your body allowed you to get rid of the extra magnesium instead of using it up. This test isn't foolproof and requires two doctor visits. Moreover, it can be hard to find a facility that actually administers magnesium tolerance tests.

Even though a magnesium tolerance test can give you the best available idea of what your magnesium status is, no single method is considered the gold standard. Magnesium tolerance tests aren't typically taken, because a clinical evaluation (in which a doctor or professional analyzes your signs and symptoms) is typically required to diagnose a deficiency. If you're extremely opposed to supplementing without a test, ask your doctor about getting a magnesium tolerance test. But even if you do that, he or she might suggest just trying a supplement for a month or two to see how it affects your health. The good news is that magnesium is relatively safe (and inexpensive!), so supplementing with it to see if you notice a difference in your symptoms is typically a good option as long as you've talked to your doctor first.

And so, the answer to the question "Do I really need to take magnesium?" is actually simple and complicated at the same time. The simple answer is, "Yes, probably." But the long answer is that magnesium tests are rarely done to determine if a person has an actual, clinical magnesium deficiency, and oftentimes deficiencies are diagnosed by just trying out a supplement or assessing symptoms and lifestyle factors that might put you at risk.

## SIGNS YOU HAVE A MAGNESIUM DEFICIENCY

As we just learned, getting tested for a magnesium deficiency isn't a simple process. And surprise! Neither is identifying signs and symptoms of a deficiency. Because of magnesium's diverse activities in the human body, deficiencies present with a wide variety of signs and symptoms that also overlap with other conditions. According to leading integrative and functional medicine doctors, there are some common symptoms that reveal you may not be getting quite as much magnesium as you should be. These are:

- Muscle cramping, weakness, fatigue, twitching
- Insomnia
- Irritability
- Sensitivity to loud noises
- Anxiety

- Autism
- Depression
- ADD/ADHD
- Asthma
- Palpitations
- Osteoporosis
- Recurrent bacterial or fungal infections due to low levels of nitric oxide or a depressed immune system
- Tooth cavities
- Impotence
- Eclampsia and preeclampsia
- Angina
- Restless leg syndrome
- Worsened PMS symptoms
- Behavioral disorders and mood swings
- Constipation
- Anal spasms
- Headaches
- Migraines
- Fibromyalgia
- Chronic fatigue
- Asthma
- Kidney stones
- Diabetes
- Obesity
- High blood pressure
- Thyroid disorders
- PMS, especially menstrual cramps
- Irritable bladder
- Irritable bowel syndrome and other gut disorders
- Reflux

Now, I want you to take all of these with a grain of salt—the quality of the research varies greatly when it comes to whether or not these symptoms are strongly related to magnesium deficiency. Instead, I want you to pay close attention to the general category that many of the items on this list fall into. You'll notice that many of them qualify as "hyperirritability" disorders—which occur when the nervous system or another part of the body is overly active, resonating in symptoms such as cramps, headaches, spasms, irritation, inflammation, constriction, palpitations. These symptoms all seem to share an underlying root cause and magnesium could play an important role here.

## YOU MIGHT HAVE A MAGNESIUM DEFICIENCY, BUT IT'S NOT THE ANSWER TO ALL YOUR HEALTH WOES

Now, if you looked at the list of signs and symptoms of a magnesium deficiency and thought to yourself, *these could be caused by any number of things*, I totally get it. It makes no sense to claim that a complex and widespread condition like obesity, which plagues millions of people in the world, is caused by a simple magnesium deficiency. I'm definitely not here to tell you that all these conditions could be cured by taking magnesium. That would be crazy.

I do, however, urge you to take a closer look at complex conditions such as obesity and diabetes and realize that they are just as I said: complex. Neither one is caused by one thing but by a wild and crazy combination of insufficiencies and dysfunctions. Take obesity, for example: In recent years we've learned that weight gain isn't just about eating more calories than you're burning; and it's not just about genetic or environmental factors, either. Obesity has everything to do with how our metabolism is working, how well we're absorbing nutrients, which nutrients we're eating, how healthy our microbiome is, how balanced our blood sugar is, what our sleep quality is like, how stressed we are (the list, quite literally, could go on and on). When you think about it this way, if a magnesium supplement was able to improve just one or two of the factors playing a role in obesity, would it be of value or worth studying more and experimenting with, assuming that it's safe? I think so.

I've been working in the integrative health and wellness industry for a while now, and one of the things I find frustrating on almost a daily basis is how we spend way too much time looking for one solution to or underlying cause of our health issues. "Maybe it's Lyme disease, or chronic fatigue, or celiac disease," I hear so many of my friends and colleagues say. And while there are rare cases of someone feeling sick and finally figuring out that it can be attributed to one solitary root cause, more often than not, that's not the case at all. So how do most people get healthy again? The majority of the people I know who have turned their health around have done so by making small healthy changes, one by one, that eventually snowball (in a good way) into better health.

It's ultimately up to you to decide if you might benefit from a little extra magnesium, but the good news is that supplementing with magnesium at normal dosages is generally considered safe and is also—huge bonus—inexpensive. So really, sometimes the easiest way to determine whether or not you'll benefit from magnesium is just to give it a try. When I asked Dr. Will Cole, a functional medicine expert and author of the book *Ketotarian,* whether or not everyone needs a magnesium supplement, his response was: "I think everyone can benefit from some extra magnesium. Even if it's just for the relaxation benefits alone—everyone can use that at some point. A lack of magnesium is associated with many other symptoms including cramps, brain fog, anxiety, inflammation, and diabetes as well." Curious about what other conditions magnesium might help with and how it works? That's what the next chapter is all about. Onward!

# The Health Benefits of Magnesium

If you've read up on the health benefits of magnesium, you already know that there are a ton of claims out there about its ability to help with dozens of different conditions. You've probably heard it paired with words like "healed," "cured," and ... actually, I'm going to stop myself right there because this should already be setting off some major red flags. I'm a big believer in magnesium as a tool (a powerful tool, even) for better health, but it's important to take each benefit of magnesium at face value and to evaluate the research that exists to back it up. Each and every claim about magnesium is accompanied by varying levels of scientific support, which can range anywhere from anecdotal evidence (that is, people use it and they think it works) to randomized, double-blind, placebo-controlled studies, which are considered the gold standard of scientific research.

This chapter covers most (but not all) of the many different benefits of magnesium. It focuses on the benefits that have peer-reviewed research or strong clinical observation to support them and are the most applicable to the typical health-conscious individuals who are curious about magnesium, how it works, and how they might benefit from it. It's good to be skeptical, of course. But now that we know what a crucial role magnesium plays in so many biological functions (thanks to Chapter 1), it makes more sense that it shows promise for treating such a wide range of diseases, disorders, and everyday health woes.

## MAGNESIUM AND PAIN

Of all the benefits of magnesium, the possibility of treating various types of pain are some of the most exciting. Magnesium has shown promise for treating many different types of pain, including those related to nerve and muscle dysfunction and the symptoms they create, such as pain, spasms, and tension.

So how can magnesium potentially reduce pain? A large portion of magnesium's pain-reducing qualities can be attributed to its ability to help muscles relax; it plays a central role in muscle contraction—but that's not the only reason! Magnesium can also interact with NMDA (N-methyl-D-aspartate) receptors in the brain, which play an important role in nerve pain. Research has suggested that magnesium could contribute to easing nerve pain related to pancreatic cancer, and it has also shown promise for managing pain related to fibromyalgia, which is an autoimmune condition characterized by widespread muscle pain and tenderness. Researchers also postulate that a magnesium deficiency might be a major amplifier of pain in general. In other words, if you're deficient in magnesium, whatever pain you have might be worse because of the deficiency.

It can sometimes be difficult to wrap your mind around magnesium's ability to not only reduce minor aches and pains from, say, a long day at work or a hard workout at the gym but also its potential for treating serious conditions characterized by chronic pain. Can it really do both? What I've learned is that the answer depends on what role magnesium played in the pain to begin with. Correcting a magnesium deficiency might help reduce pain, but someone with healthy levels of magnesium that's suffering from pain for another reason might not see those results.

After learning that there is, indeed, a pretty strong link between magnesium and pain relief, you might wonder why it's not always a consideration when someone is struggling with pain. This is especially true when you learn that the scientific community has been aware of this connection for decades. The authors of a study published in *Canadian Family Physician* in 1996 wrote, "Magnesium deficiency should always be included in the differential diagnosis of patients who present with persistent or severe muscle pain." That article was written more than 20 years ago, yet it's still not considered standard protocol to consider magnesium when someone is suffering from pain, even when the alternative existing treatments, including opioids, are extremely addictive and come with a host of side effects such as constipation, nausea, and drowsiness. I shudder to think about the number of people suffering right now whose magnesium deficiencies are being overlooked. There are still a lot of questions to be answered about the correlation between magnesium and pain management, but it's well worth exploring.

## MAGNESIUM AND HEADACHES

It would have been easy enough to classify headaches and migraines under the umbrella of general pain. But because there is a large number of people using magnesium to treat headaches and migraines specifically, they deserve their own section. Many studies have connected migraines and headaches of all kinds to a deficiency in magnesium. Research also supports the idea that daily supplementation with magnesium can help prevent migraines, especially those related to PMS. In one study, patients received 600 mg of magnesium citrate. After 9 to 12 weeks, their headache frequency was reduced by 41.6 percent compared to the placebo group whose headache frequency was reduced by 15.8 percent. You might be surprised by a 600 mg dosage as that's almost double what the RDA suggests for magnesium. If you're suffering from headaches or migraines, it's important to talk to your doctor about dosing magnesium and which form will be best for your specific situation.

Holistic and conventional doctors alike often use IV magnesium to help fend off migraines, and it's pretty successful. Dr. Ilene Ruhoy, an integrative neurologist who is one of my go-to experts on all things brain health, is one of them. She often suggests IV magnesium for her patients' migraines. When I asked her why it works, she explained:

"Magnesium deficiency has been associated with cerebral hyperexcitability, which is thought to contribute to both migraines and seizures. Magnesium sulfate given intravenously can be very effective for status migrainosus, which is a migraine that is refractory to multiple abortive treatments. This can be obtained at most urgent care centers, emergency departments, but also headache clinics." This treatment option for migraines seems to become more popular by the day.

Supplementing with magnesium might not be the magic cure for your headaches or migraines, but it could be one more thing that allows you to stay below your unique headache threshold. Not to mention, when you compare the side effects of magnesium to those of migraine medications—as many as two-thirds of migraine sufferers avoid their prescription medication because of side effects such as fatigue, muscle weakness, chest pressure, racing heartbeat, nausea, and difficulty thinking—magnesium seems like an even more attractive option.

## MAGNESIUM AND ANXIETY

As I mentioned in Chapter 2, magnesium plays an important part in our nervous system health and in our stress and relaxation responses. It's no surprise, then, that people report magnesium is helpful for managing their anxiety; in fact, anxiety is one of the most common reasons why people take magnesium. According to Anxiety and Depression Association of America, 1 in 14 people worldwide suffers from an anxiety disorder. This includes anything from a generalized anxiety disorder and panic disorders to agoraphobia, social anxiety disorder, and phobias. Sadly, existing medications for anxiety-related mental health conditions can be addictive and come with debilitating side effects. This means there's a lot of demand for tools that can help the millions of people to cope with anxiety in a way that doesn't cause as many problems as the anxiety itself.

We're still learning the exact mechanisms by which magnesium helps keep anxiety at bay, but we know it affects neuronal receptors, key neurotransmitters, and hormonal activity in key areas of the brain. For instance, magnesium is an important cofactor in the creation of serotonin and dopamine, which are two neurotransmitters that perform very important functions in mood and relaxation. Magnesium also influences the activity of GABA (gamma-Aminobutyric acid, or γ-aminobutyric acid), the main inhibitory neurotransmitter in the brain that is intricately involved in anxiety (GABA receptors are actually the target of benzodiazepines such as Xanax, which is the most popular class of drug for anxiety). Both animal and human studies show that there's a correlation between low levels of magnesium and an increase in stress and mood disorders. We should also remember that it's suspected that in periods of extreme stress, magnesium is used up by the body more quickly, leaving us vulnerable to a deficiency. Magnesium has also been shown to improve symptoms of depression and other mental health conditions such as mania, which makes sense when you consider that many mental health conditions involve similar pathways in the brain and are intricately connected.

All that said, none of the research on magnesium and anxiety, or any mental health condition for that matter, is conclusive. Personally, I don't notice any immediate change in my anxiety levels when I take magnesium as a capsule or supplement, but I do notice an immediate difference when I make the time to get in the tub for an Epsom salt bath or give myself a nice magnesium oil foot rub (or check out my End-of-Day

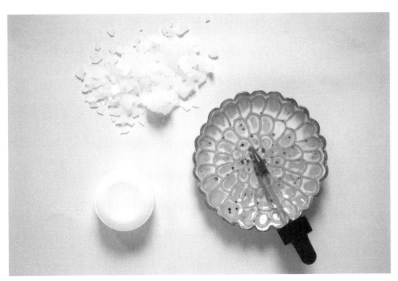

Foot Soak on page 131 ). I also feel a difference in my stress levels and anxiety when I've taken magnesium very regularly over a long period of time. It's hard to pinpoint whether or not the changes I notice can be directly attributed to magnesium alone, but knowing what role it plays in the nervous system and relaxation response, it makes sense that I'd see these benefits.

## MAGNESIUM AND CHRONIC FATIGUE

More than a million people in America suffer from chronic fatigue, which affects more women than men and manifests as extreme tiredness and loss of energy and motivation. Chronic fatigue is one of those illnesses that conventional medicine isn't sure what to do with or how to treat, which makes it a common entry point into the world of alternative medicine. Oftentimes, magnesium is a key player in holistic treatment plans for chronic fatigue. Remember when we talked about magnesium playing a role in hundreds of biochemical reactions in the body? Well, a lot of them have to do with energy production.

"Energy production" really means the processes occurring in our bodies that turn food into usable energy. When we eat a meal, the fats and carbs and proteins we eat don't just turn into instant energy. Our body has to break them down into smaller, more workable pieces, absorb them, and then send them to specific locations where they can be used. When what you've eaten finally reaches your cells, it's transformed into ATP (adenosine triphosphate)—which is basically like an energy currency the body uses to fuel you—in tiny cellular structures called the mitochondria. This process of turning food into ATP requires magnesium. In particular, magnesium is needed by the proteins that synthesize ATP in the mitochondria. If you had any further doubts that magnesium plays an important role in our body's energy levels, you should know that ATP is often found in the form MgATP, which is just ATP bound to magnesium.

Studies have pointed out that chronic fatigue—and other illnesses characterized by extreme fatigue—are somehow related to low levels of magnesium. Magnesium is one of the most commonly recommended supplements for this group of disorders. One study that tested magnesium malate on fibromyalgia patients for eight weeks showed a "critical role for magnesium and malate in ATP production under aerobic and hypoxic conditions; and indirect evidence for magnesium and malate deficiency." There is also a seriously suspicious overlap in symptoms between chronic fatigue and magnesium deficiency. Unfortunately, many of these studies were published a long time ago. We are in serious need of up-to-date research and clinical trials regarding the link between magnesium and chronic fatigue.

One last thing: I'll talk about this in-depth a little later on, but I'm not a huge fan of IV supplements—especially from these IV infusion cafes that are popping up, as I think they send the wrong message about when and how IV supplementation should be used (that is, not for alieving hangovers). But I can say that if I was suffering from a mysterious and debilitating illness such as chronic fatigue and I was in a place in my life where I felt I could afford them, this is one situation where I would consider trying IV supplements. My reasoning is pretty simple: It's by far the most bioavailable form of a nutrient and it's fast-acting, which means you'd know if it was working more quickly than you would if you were taking magnesium orally or topically.

## MAGNESIUM AND ATHLETIC PERFORMANCE AND RECOVERY

Listen up all athletes and dedicated gym goers! It's nice to take a break from talking about illness and disease and instead to discuss how to use magnesium to optimize health and boost athletic performance. Interestingly, magnesium does this through many of the mechanisms we've already talked about, those that help our bodies produce energy and reduce pain. Epsom salts have long been used to help athletes recover from strenuous exercise, which—as anyone who's ever taken a Barry's Bootcamp class knows—can cause a lot of joint and muscle pain and stiffness.

But what does the research say? Studies have shown that a magnesium deficiency can impair athletic performance and might also increase the negative consequences of strenuous and intense exercise on the body. Plus, a deficiency in magnesium has been related to an increase in lactic acid buildup, which could also help explain why it seems to be so beneficial post-workout.

This connection is especially relevant for those taking NSAIDs (non-steroidal anti-inflammatory drugs) or other over-the-counter meds to recover from their workouts. If you're a high-performance athlete or a huge gym fanatic, an Epsom salt bath could be your new secret weapon for optimizing performance and for making your workouts a little easier on your body. To really up the ante, try pairing the Electrolyte Recovery Drink recipe (page 110) with the Post-Workout Bath (page 151). Ah, sweet, sweet relaxation.

## MAGNESIUM AND INFLAMMATION

If you've read my other book, *CBD Oil: Everyday Secrets,* you know at least a few things about the inflammatory response, inflammation, and autoimmunity. You also know what a massive role inflammation plays in our health and how we can use lifestyle changes—including CBD!—to help quell it. Magnesium doesn't have quite the same relationship with inflammation that CBD does, but there are definitely some important connections worth talking about.

For starters, studies have shown that low levels of magnesium in the blood are linked to higher levels of inflammation in the body. The researchers of one study concluded: "Subclinical magnesium deficiency caused by low dietary intake often occurring in the population is a predisposing factor for chronic inflammatory stress that is conducive for chronic disease." Another randomized, double-blind placebo-controlled trial showed that oral magnesium supplementation decreases C-reactive protein levels in people with prediabetes and magnesium deficiency. Measuring C-reactive protein levels is one of the most commonly measured inflammatory markers, and it is a good way to determine whether or not someone is suffering from chronic inflammation.

It's also been suggested that on a cellular level, magnesium actually decreases inflammation. In fact, inflammation might be the thing that connects magnesium deficiency to many of the illnesses discussed in this book. One study concluded that "further studies are still needed to assess more accurately the role of magnesium in the immune response in humans, but these experimental findings in animal models suggest that inflammation is the missing link to explain the role of magnesium in many pathological conditions."

The take-home? If you suffer from chronic inflammation, an inflammatory disease, or an autoimmune disease, supplementing with magnesium—along with other inflammation-reducing lifestyle changes such as reducing your intake of sugar, alcohol, and refined carbs—is worth exploring.

## MAGNESIUM AND INSOMNIA

There's no doubt that America has a sleep problem. People aren't sleeping enough, they aren't sleeping soundly, and they're suffering from insomnia, sleep apnea, and any number of other sleep disorders. Improving sleep is tough and requires us to overcome both personal health issues and societal pressures to do more and sleep less. So can magnesium help? It looks promising. One study, in particular, showed that magnesium supplementation can lead to an increase in sleep time and an easier time falling asleep compared to a placebo. The same study also showed lower levels of cortisol (the stress hormone) and higher levels of melatonin—the hormone we start producing when the sun goes down to signal to our body that it's time to unwind—in those taking magnesium.

But what are the mechanisms behind this? When it comes to magnesium and sleep, there are several factors at play; we've discussed a few of them already. The role magnesium plays in muscle relaxation might be one reason why it seems to help with sleep, because we need to relax our muscles before we're able to actually drift off. In addition, magnesium interacts with both NMDA receptors (antagonists of which are linked to improved sleep and relaxation as well as nerve pain, which we learned before) and GABA receptors (remember, this is the neurotransmitter involved in quieting down nerve activity, and we learned it plays a big role in anxiety). As we learned in Chapter 2, we also know that magnesium can help stimulate the parasympathetic nervous system, which is a major hint that it can help our nervous system chill out if we're still feeling a little bit amped at the end of the day when, instead, we want to feel sleepy and ready to cozy-up.

Supplementing with magnesium has also been shown to improve insomnia related to restless leg syndrome, which is an endlessly annoying condition that causes uncomfortable sensations in the legs and an urge to move them. It's classified as both a sleep disorder and also a disorder of the nervous system because it often occurs at night when you're lying in bed. The research is very preliminary, but it's suspected that restless leg syndrome might be caused by a deficiency in magnesium. In any event, taking magnesium is a route that many people should consider before trying sleep medicines or other pharmaceuticals.

## MAGNESIUM AND DIGESTION

It's been shown over and over again that, indeed, all disease "begins in the gut," like Hippocrates wrote so many years ago. Our knowledge of the gut microbiome—which is the ecosystem of bacteria living in our GI tract—has absolutely exploded in recent years. We've learned so much about how the health of our GI tract impacts our mood, brain functioning, immune system, hormone health, energy levels, and more.

Our digestive systems are amazingly complex, and we often take them for granted. Because of this, a lot can go wrong with our health when our digestion is awry. One of the most frustrating and uncomfortable maladies is constipation. At the very least, it's annoying and uncomfortable; at its worst, chronic constipation can be complicated by anal fissures, hemorrhoids, or even fecal impaction—which are not things you ever want to experience if you can help it. Eating more fiber, drinking plenty of water, and getting enough exercise can all help fend off chronic constipation, but they don't work for everyone all the time. It's easy enough to turn to over-the-counter remedies for quick relief, but if constipation is a chronic problem for you it's wise to take a more proactive approach.

So can magnesium help? It sure can. In fact, this is one of the most well-established and scientifically supported benefits of magnesium. For example, in a 2014 double-blind placebo-controlled trial on 244 adult women with functional constipation, magnesium supplementation led to an improved number of stools. Magnesium seems to be a great option for daily supplementation for those who suffer from chronic slow digestion, and it is virtually side-effect free when taken at appropriate doses. Just be careful, because higher doses of magnesium and certain types of magnesium are known to cause diarrhea and GI distress—so it is possible to overdo it. Magnesium often gets a bad rap for causing digestive distress, but if you take it in the right dose it should be pretty gentle and won't cause you to run urgently to the bathroom.

How does magnesium work to treat occasional constipation? Certain types of magnesium (like magnesium citrate) are osmotic laxatives. That means they pull water into your intestines from your body and relax your bowels to soften things up and to get them moving. Magnesium is even prescribed by doctors before colonoscopies and other procedures that require empty bowels.

## MAGNESIUM AND PERIOD-RELATED HEALTH WOES

Hey ladies! When it comes to our monthly cycle, magnesium has a lot of potential for the full gamut of symptoms. So whether you experience mild symptoms (lucky you) or barely survive the full-blown hormone roller coaster every month, magnesium can help.

For starters, there's reason to believe that magnesium can help alleviate premenstrual symptoms of fluid retention such as weight gain, swelling of extremities, breast tenderness, and abdominal bloating. And if you're someone who relies on over-the-counter medications a few days a month (or more!) for cramps, you'll be happy to learn that a review of existing clinical trials showed that magnesium supplements provided relief from painful cramping during menses without any significant adverse events. An Epsom salt bath is also an excellent choice; on page 155, a recipe called Hormone-Balancing Bath features magnesium with clary sage and chamomile, two essential oils that are great for female hormone balance and relaxation.

## MAGNESIUM AND HEART HEALTH

Poor heart health has been the leading cause of death in America for almost 100 years, with most heart conditions directly linked to lifestyle factors such as smoking, lack of exercise, and the standard American diet, which is high in saturated fats and inflammatory foods. I want to start off this section by saying that if you're suffering from a chronic illness of any sort, including heart disease, you should always talk to your doctor before making any drastic changes. Although there is a close connection between magnesium and heart health, you shouldn't be making any decisions about your heart health alone.

Now that we have that behind us, research has connected low levels of magnesium to heart issues, including blood pressure problems, arterial plaque build-up, calcification of soft tissues, cholesterol, and hardening of the arteries. Carolyn Dean, a medical doctor, naturopathic doctor, and one of the world's top experts on magnesium wrote: "The fact that low levels of magnesium are associated with all the risk factors and symptoms of heart disease, hypertension, diabetes, high cholesterol, heart arrhythmia, angina and heart attack can no longer be ignored; the evidence is much too compelling." In one example, a study with 241,378 participants published in the *American Journal of Clinical Nutrition* uncovered that a diet high in magnesium could reduce the risk of a stroke by 8 percent. A review paper also concluded that "subclinical magnesium deficiency increases the risk of numerous types of cardiovascular disease, costs nations around the world an incalculable amount of health care costs and suffering, and should be considered a public health crisis." Knowing this, you might wonder why everyone doesn't already know about the connection between magnesium status and heart health. Believe me, I've wondered the same thing.

So what's the take-home here? A magnesium supplement isn't the one and only answer to the worldwide epidemic of heart disease—we definitely still have to tackle smoking, stress, sedentary lifestyles, trans fats, and processed foods—but it appears to play an important role. Eating a magnesium-rich diet might be a viable way to prevent heart disease from occurring. If you have heart disease, especially one of the illnesses mentioned here, and your doctor dismisses you when you bring up a magnesium supplement, get a second opinion and see if another doctor says the same thing. The link between magnesium and heart disease is pretty hard to argue against, and magnesium should at least be a consideration.

## MAGNESIUM AND BONE HEALTH

Earlier I wrote about the connections between magnesium, calcium, and bone health. We learned that a *lot* of magnesium is hanging out in our bones, about 60 percent of the total magnesium in our bodies. You learned, maybe even for the first time, that you were misled when you were told that calcium was the be-all and end-all for building and maintaining strong bones.

As it turns out, magnesium, vitamin K, and vitamin $D_3$ might be even more important for bone health than calcium. In fact, one study showed that supplementing with magnesium for just one month slowed the progression of osteoporosis. A 2013 study that assessed the then-current knowledge of magnesium and bone health concluded that "overall, controlling and maintaining magnesium homeostasis represents a helpful intervention to maintaining bone integrity." In other studies, results showed that magnesium restriction promoted osteoporosis and that a low-magnesium diet negatively impacted bone health. When it was tested on animals, bones that were deficient in magnesium were more likely to be brittle and fragile.

I've been giving calcium a bad rap so far. But, interestingly, the reason why magnesium seems to help with bone formation actually has a lot to do with calcium. Magnesium stimulates the hormone calcitonin, which works to draw calcium into the bones, thereby preserving bone structure. This action has been linked to a lower risk of osteoporosis and other diseases such as arthritis, heart attacks, and kidney stones as well. As you can see, calcium is quite important; it has just been touted as the end-all, be-all for so long that other bone-health supporting nutrients were ignored.

So what does a bone-health-friendly diet look like? If you have osteoporosis, I suggest that you consult with an integrative or functional medicine doctor. But if you're simply looking to support your bones, I recommend that you focus on a whole foods diet rich in essential vitamins and minerals—especially magnesium, vitamin D, and calcium together—and low in processed foods, which have often lost essential minerals.

## MAGNESIUM AND BLOOD SUGAR BALANCE

There's no arguing that diabetes is one of the biggest health threats facing our world today. More than 30 million people in the United States have diabetes (that is 9.4 percent of the U.S. population). You might think that because you don't have diabetes, this number doesn't apply to you, but it's important to know that almost 24 percent of people with diabetes are undiagnosed. In addition, prediabetes—a condition characterized by increased thirst, frequent urination, and fatigue that eventually leads to diabetes—affects one in three Americans, although only 10 percent are aware of it.

Diabetes and prediabetes are conditions that modern conventional health care is failing to treat successfully on the individual level and is failing to control on the population level. There are many reasons for this, but a big one is that type 2 diabetes is directly related to diet and lifestyle, two things that most doctors don't get sufficient training in while they're in medical school. Did you know that the average doctor gets less than 20 hours of nutrition training in their four years of medical school? It's true. In practical terms, it means that millions of people are suffering from type 2 diabetes—a condition that, depending on the severity, can not only can be improved or managed with lifestyle changes but even reversed completely.

This is a book about magnesium, so you won't be surprised to learn that it plays an important role in blood sugar regulation. Research has shown that magnesium can help with glucose metabolism, and it therefore might be helpful for the prevention and management of type 2 diabetes. In fact, studies have suggested that dietary magnesium deficiency might actually be a direct contributor to insulin resistance.

Unfortunately, treating diabetes with lifestyle changes requires time and effort from both patient and clinician (whether it be a doctor, dietician, or other professional); it's more involved than just giving a person a magnesium supplement and a pamphlet that says to avoid soda and candy. Stabilizing blood sugar naturally requires you to take a good, hard look at your daily sugar and carbohydrate intake (including even healthy foods like rice and fruit), address your stress levels and sleep quality, and to make a very firm commitment to exercise. And for those working with integrative and functional medicine doctors, a more intensive plan may be prescribed, such as reducing or eliminating caffeine and alcohol, going gluten free, and cutting down on snacking.

All that said, it can be done! I've never been diagnosed with prediabetes or diabetes, but I do have a history of pretty intense "hanger" (hungry-anger) and always used to get nauseous if I hadn't eaten in more than three hours or so. After following the recommendations of leading holistic doctors for a few years (many of the same recommendations they'd suggest to prediabetics), I'm happy to report that I'm no longer someone who gets tired, shaky, or nauseous between meals or has to carry a granola bar with me everywhere I go. Magnesium is just one of many blood-sugar-balancing ingredients that I incorporate into my routine. If you need some inspiration, check out the recipe for Blood-Sugar-Balancing Cinnamon Bites on page 104.

## MAGNESIUM AND WEIGHT LOSS AND MANAGEMENT

Now that you know magnesium plays an important role in diabetes prevention and healthy blood sugar regulation, it probably won't surprise you to learn that it also plays an important role in weight management and the prevention of obesity and metabolic syndrome. Metabolic syndrome is a condition characterized by high blood pressure, high blood sugar, excess visceral fat, abnormal cholesterol, and blood lipid levels that increase your risk of obesity and obesity-related conditions such as heart disease, diabetes, and stroke. Put simply, it's the name given to the many dysfunctions that start to occur in the body when a person's unhealthy lifestyle starts to catch up with them.

Several studies, including one published in the *Journal of the American Heart Association,* have found that a diet rich in magnesium helps protect against metabolic syndrome. One even found that women with the highest intake of dietary magnesium had a 27-percent-lower incidence of metabolic syndrome, which is a pretty shocking number. If you're struggling with your weight or any of these weight-related conditions, it's a good idea to make sure your diet is rich in all the important nutrients—especially magnesium. Luckily, magnesium-rich foods are some of the healthiest foods on the planet and many of them help you maintain a healthy weight. Some of these include leafy greens (chock-full of vitamins and minerals), nuts (which make a great, healthy snack), and fish (which is super filling and great for your heart health). If you're looking to jump-start weight loss or to increase your chances of fending off metabolic syndrome, incorporating some of the recipes in this book into your daily routine may help you get there.

I think it's safe to say that the list of conditions that are associated with low levels of magnesium—or might benefit from magnesium supplementation—*is very long.* And while we've covered many of the most relevant ones, magnesium might also benefit people with asthma—by relaxing the bronchioles of the lungs—ADHD, and even cancer. Epidemiological studies point to magnesium deficiency as a risk factor for certain cancers, and having a magnesium deficiency can potentially interfere with or complicate cancer treatment.

You might have already noticed that many of the conditions noted in this chapter are more common in women than men—including auto-immune disease, anxiety, osteoporosis, and the obvious ones like menstrual cramps and mood swings related to hormonal fluctuations. So do women need to supplement with magnesium more often than men? Are women at greater risk for a deficiency? It's possible, especially because some of the things that deplete the body of magnesium—like anxiety and the use of certain medications—are more common among women.

And this brings me to an important point: Ladies, for whatever reason, we're at a higher risk of developing certain conditions and deficiencies, and so it's important to know that your health care is a little bit different for you than it is for men. Did you know that women are both more likely to use the health care system in general and more likely to explore alternative treatments? They are also, historically speaking, the gatekeepers for the health of their family unit—they are usually in charge of things like nutrition and hours of sleep. But despite being the center of family health, women have long been neglected and ignored by the health care industry. What do I mean by this? For starters, the male body has always been the model for treatment, and men are way overrepresented in medical research. This means that most drugs and treatments have been developed to work in the male body and then just adapted to female bodies after the fact. Men also experience shorter wait times in the ER and are more likely to have their symptoms taken seriously by doctors. For example, if a man and a woman both go to the ER with chest pains, the man is more likely to be evaluated right away for a potential heart attack and the woman is more likely to be dismissed as having a panic attack. Ugh.

Here's what I want you to take away from this: If you're a woman, you might have to be a little more assertive in order to make sure you're getting high-quality care. Keep that information in mind whenever you go to the doctor, *especially if it's an emergency situation*. Also, keep this in mind if you're suffering from something like chronic fatigue or adrenal fatigue or any condition that presents with a wide range of vague symptoms that are hard to categorize. They can often be brushed off by doctors, and this will be even truer if you are a woman. Don't ever let someone tell you there's no reason why you're not feeling your best, and always get a second opinion if you don't feel satisfied.

# 6

# How to Choose a Magnesium Supplement

Now that you're well versed in the science of magnesium, you're probably ready to track down a supplement and to give it a try. At this stage, you'll be confronted with a lot of different options, and honestly, this part of the process can be overwhelming. It's not just the brand of magnesium to consider but also the dose, the form, and the delivery method. In other words: How in the world do you choose between the magnesium foot spray or the supplement capsule or the drink? And then how do you choose between the endless brand options for each?

In recent years, the supplement industry has ballooned. And while it's nice to have options, the downside is that you have a ton of different brands all claiming that their product is the best—that they're the most responsible, transparent, and effective. In a perfect world, only the high-quality supplements would get the spotlight, but unfortunately, marketing and attractive packaging tend to go a long way in driving customers to purchase products without looking carefully enough at the ingredients list. My goal for this chapter is to leave you with a set of skills that will help you sort through the junk so that you can choose a product that really fits your needs.

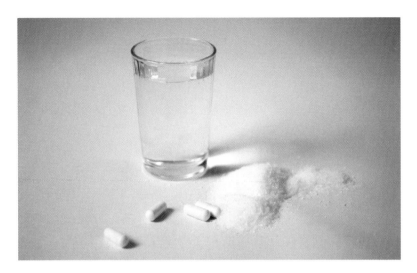

## HOW SUPPLEMENTS ARE REGULATED (OR NOT REGULATED)

It's not uncommon for people to exclaim that the supplement industry is *completely unregulated,* but that's not entirely true. The Food and Drug Administration (FDA) and the Federal Trade Commission (FTC) are in charge of overseeing supplements, but it's done in a way that is, for lack of a better word, strange. Here's what I mean:

In 1994, a law called the Dietary Supplement Health and Education Act of 1994 (also referred to as DSHEA) officially set the standard for supplement regulations. This law required that supplements—which are defined as dietary ingredients, including vitamins, minerals, amino acids, and herbs or botanicals, as well as other substances that can be used to supplement the diet—be regulated more like foods than drugs. Prior to this law, there was a lot of debate about how to classify supplements: Do they need to be approved by the FDA before they're sold, and should consumers have to get them through a health care provider?

There was quite a bit of drama surrounding this issue, and at one point the government tried to regulate supplements much more closely. In response, *thousands* of people called Congress to protest (in fact, more people called their representatives about this issue than about the Vietnam War), and the public made it very clear that they didn't want pharmacists, doctors, or the government to be heavily involved in the world of vitamins, minerals, and herbs. And so, DSHEA was passed. The upside of this law is that it provides access for everyone, but the downside is that it mostly leaves the public to fend for itself in terms of assessing quality and safety.

And so when people call the industry "unregulated," what they really mean is that supplements on the shelves have *not* been tested and approved by the FDA for safety, purity, or quality. The FDA does involve itself by setting good manufacturing practices (GMPs), which require a company to properly identify the materials in their supplements, register with the FDA, and keep detailed batch records. But really, these requirements are the absolute bare minimum and don't stop bad (or even dangerous) supplements from reaching the shelves. Periodically, the FDA will check in on supplement companies to make sure they're following these basic rules, but they only really investigate further when there's a bad apple—such as a company that makes egregiously unfounded claims (like their supplement can cure a disease or help you lose 20 pounds in three days, for example) or when there is a contaminant in the product or when a product contains an ingredient that's causing harm. Basically, the burden of proof is on the FDA to show that something is *unsafe,* instead of on the company to prove its product is safe *before* it hits the shelves. This means that when you buy a supplement you're putting your health in the hands of the company that made the product.

## HOW TO FIND A HIGH-QUALITY SUPPLEMENT: QUESTIONS TO ASK BEFORE YOU BUY

All that said, there are definitely companies that set their own high standards. They do this by getting the quality, purity, and safety of their products tested by in-house labs and/or third-party labs that follow ISO (International Organization for Standardization) certified procedures, which is the standard that defines the requirements for a lab's processes and management. This isn't required by law, but it's a sign that the company is jumping through extra hoops to make sure that what they print on the label is actually what they put in the bottle. This means that there is a way for you to take supplements and to feel very secure in what you're getting. You just have to be a savvy consumer who is able to tell what's what.

So how do you tell what's what? Well, that depends on what kind of supplement you're looking for in the first place—whether it be magnesium, echinacea, vitamin D, or something else. First, I'll go over some general supplement-buying guidelines and then I'll move on to some magnesium-specific ones. When it comes to buying supplements in general, there are some basic rules to follow, and they typically come in the form of questions that you should be able to answer by looking at the label, scanning a product or company website, or dialing a company's customer service department for a quick phone call (a novel idea in 2019, I know!).

- **What can the supplement company tell you about its sourcing?** In other words, can they tell you about the farm where the herb was grown and describe their practices? Do they know which lake the spirulina is sourced from? Can they tell you which animals their collagen is derived from and if they were grass-fed/free-range? These are all highly important questions and can mean the difference between a great supplement and a not-so-great one.
- **Does the supplement company encourage you to work with a health care practitioner?** There are interactions, dosage information, and contraindications that you should definitely be aware of—especially if you have a chronic health condition of some kind or are taking medications. It's a good sign when health care providers use the products from a particular company and encourage you to buy supplements from that company through them, as opposed to advising you to self-prescribe and go it alone. This might mean less direct business for the company, but it's the responsible thing to do.
- **Is the supplement company making claims that sound too good to be true?** Some red flags are words like "cure," "miracle," and anything that's marketed for "weight loss" or "male enhancement." You want to make sure your supplement isn't promising you something it never planned to deliver. There have even been reports of supplement companies slipping phar-

maceutical drugs into their supplements to make these claims seem to be true—yikes.

- **Is the supplement company investing time and money in research?** This question probably won't apply to smaller supplement companies, but it's really important for the big ones. I mean, why wouldn't a company want to help fund research or to partner with a research institution to progress scientific knowledge on their products? It's a great sign if they are investing in these endeavors, and it's worth taking pause if a big supplement company hasn't made science a priority.

- **Are they using the most bioavailable form and a therapeutic dose of the nutrient?** In other words: Are they using a form and an amount of the nutrient that will actually make a difference in your health? A great example of this is vitamin D, which you'll see on supplement labels in the form of $D_3$ and $D_2$. Many studies have shown that $D_3$ is more effective than $D_2$ and that a therapeutic dose is considered to be around 1,000 IU (international units). So, if you see a vitamin D product that is using less than 1,000 IUs or is using $D_2$, then you know it's probably not what you're looking for.

- **Do you know what (all of) the ingredients are?** One of the most important sections on a supplement label is the "additional ingredients" list. A lot of the time, this is where the list of unnecessary ingredients such as artificial colors, flavors, sugars, preservatives, and fillers is hiding. Ideally, there shouldn't be anything in your supplement that isn't there for a specific reason. When reviewing a list of things that shouldn't be in your supplement, what should you look for? Start with wheat, gluten, egg, coatings, shellacs, GMOs, magnesium stearate, trans fats, hydrogenated oils, artificial colors, flavors, and sweeteners, high-fructose corn syrup, MSG, propylene glycol, BHT, BHA, talc and other unnecessary binders, fillers (like rice flour), and preservatives.

- **Do they already have—or are they working toward—a third-party certification?** Some supplement companies will request an independent organization to evaluate the company's products for safety and quality. Such evaluations include testing for heavy metal contamination, microbes, and pesticides and other chemicals. Normally, a supplement that has been third-party tested will have an NSF (National Sanitation Foundation) sticker right on the label. Companies have to pay for this, so smaller companies won't always have it. Some larger companies will actually test their products in their own high-tech labs (which can sometimes allow for more advanced, stricter testing than what is used by a third-party lab). The take-home here is to make sure that the company knows the ins and outs of their testing process, and that it is doing their best to go above and beyond. It's a great sign if the company offers tours of their manufacturing facility.

- **Does your supplement have a "best before" or "use by" date?** The potency of many supplements decreases over time, but not all supplements have an expiration date listed on the packaging (the FDA doesn't require it). It's important to look for supplements that do show expiration dates on the packaging, because that means the company has voluntarily guaranteed the supplement's potency until that date. Also be sure to follow instructions stated on the package for proper storage and suggested use so that you get the most out of your purchase.

If you're still left with questions about your supplements or want nutrient-specific recommendations, check out the National Institutes of Health Office of Dietary Supplements (ods.od.nih.gov). Some specific brands that I'm loyal to are Thorne, Gaia Herbs, and Pure Encapsulations. I also think NOW Foods offers good value at a lower price point than the others, so they're an option if you're on a budget. You can also check out the Consumer Lab website (www.consumerlab.com)— this organization independently tests supplements for quality and then gives them a pass-or-fail score.

## HOW TO CHOOSE A MAGNESIUM SUPPLEMENT

The previous section might have been more information than you bargained for, but it's all important stuff to know! The supplement industry

Why don't we just take magnesium straight-up? Well, magnesium isn't stable and the body doesn't absorb it well when it's on its own, so we have to combine it with other substances such as salts, acids, or amino acid chelates (which are the building blocks of proteins). This is why you won't ever see just magnesium on a supplement label; instead, you'll see longer words like "magnesium citrate" or "magnesium malate." Both the size and function of the molecule that magnesium is bound to influences how well our bodies can absorb it and also which side effects (positive and negative) we might experience after taking it. The facts panel on the back of your supplement packaging will declare the amount of elemental magnesium in the product, not the weight of the entire compound. This means, for example, you don't need to worry about how much magnesium is in magnesium malate versus magnesium citrate. This makes it easier to understand dosages (no math required) and explains why there are sometimes variations in the serving sizes among brands, be it the number of capsules you need to take or scoops of a powder you are directed to use.

gets a lot of criticism, and it's not that surprising. There's a lot of noise and misinformation out there, and a lot of people out there make claims of transparency and quality when their actions and actual values tell a different story. My prediction is that in the coming years we, as consumers, will be weeding out a lot of subpar supplement companies and rewarding the ones who really have our health in mind.

So are you ready for some magnesium-specific supplement recommendations? When it comes to magnesium, not all forms are created equal, and integrative and functional medicine practitioners will recommend specific forms of magnesium for specific conditions. Seeing a supplement-savvy health care provider can help you choose the right magnesium supplement, but here are some of the common supplements you'll find and their pros and cons:

**Magnesium Glycinate:** I put magnesium glycinate first because this type of magnesium is highly absorbable and is what many people consider to be the "gold standard" of magnesium supplements. It's unlikely to cause any digestive upset at normal doses. This type of magnesium comes in powder, liquid, and pill form and is bound to glycine, which is thought to help promote sleep—making this the commonly recommended type of magnesium for insomnia. This type of magnesium is a good bet and is one of the most commonly recommended by integrative and functional medicine doctors. A drawback is that it's not the best magnesium for constipation, because it doesn't have the same laxative effects as other forms.

**Magnesium Malate:** Magnesium malate is magnesium mixed with malic acid, a compound found naturally in apples and other plant-based foods. Malic acid is known across the industry to soothe muscle pain and to help with your body's natural energy production. Specifically, fibromyalgia patients have found this type of magnesium helpful, which isn't surprising as this condition is characterized by pain and fatigue. This is a good choice if you're looking for a basic magnesium supplement, and it gives you the additional benefits from the malic acid.

**Magnesium Citrate:** This is a well-absorbed form of magnesium that is combined with citric acid, which also occurs naturally in fruits, veggies, and other foods. Magnesium citrate is popular for muscle relax-

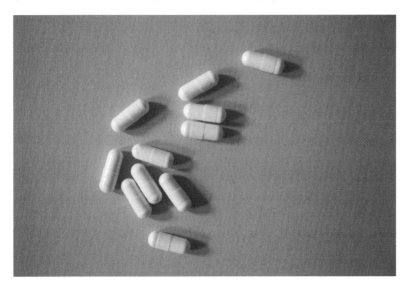

ation, cramping, and digestion. At higher doses it can cause diarrhea, but in general it's a good choice for keeping you regular if you take the right amount for your body. This is a great source of magnesium, and I like to bring magnesium citrate with me when I'm traveling and want to make sure my digestion stays in tip-top shape.

**Magnesium Oxide:** Magnesium oxide is one of the cheaper forms of magnesium, but the body does not absorb it well. If you take it in the right dose, this type of magnesium can help keep your digestion moving if you tend to get backed up, but if you take too much, magnesium oxide is famous for causing diarrhea. In general, there are better options than magnesium oxide, and it's not commonly recommended by experts unless the patient is extremely restricted when it comes to price.

**Magnesium Threonate:** Magnesium threonate is a type of magnesium known specifically for supporting brain and nervous system health. It's thought to support memory retention and learning as well as to prevent neurodegeneration and cognitive decline because of its ability to pass through the blood-brain barrier. It's not seen as often as magnesium citrate and glycinate, but if you're working with a professional and you're taking magnesium for specific brain and nervous system reasons, they might recommend it.

**Magnesium Orotate:** This is orotic acid paired up with magnesium, and this form of magnesium is sometimes hailed as the ultimate form for improving athletic performance and heart health. Although some research has supported the idea of using orotic acid for heart health, minerals bound to orotic acid don't appear to be absorbed any better than others, and there are even some questions being raised about the safety of orotic acid. This form of magnesium is also expensive, so I'd stick to magnesium citrate, glycinate, or malate.

**Magnesium Sulphate:** Magnesium sulfate is probably the most popular type of magnesium as it's what Epsom salts are made of. Magnesium sulfate salts are thought to soothe sore muscles and to promote detox and relaxation. People have historically taken this type of magnesium internally, but it can definitely cause diarrhea so I would recommend reserving this one for use in the bathtub. Be sure to check out one of the luxurious Epsom salt bath recipes in this book to take advantage of magnesium sulfate.

**Magnesium Chloride:** Magnesium chloride solutions are commonly referred to as "magnesium oil." Interestingly, magnesium chloride is not actually an oil at all; it's just a supersaturated solution of water, magnesium, and chloride. It feels wet and oily because of its high pH. This type of magnesium is often given to people who have digestive problems that might prevent them from absorbing magnesium orally. Magnesium chloride is also available in "flakes," a solid, and a crystallized format used for baths (much like Epsom salts).

Speaking of Epsom salts and magnesium oil, it's about time I talked about transdermal magnesium and the debate over whether or not this is the best way (or even a legitimate way at all) to get your daily dose of this mineral.

## UNPACKING THE DEBATE OVER TRANSDERMAL MAGNESIUM

There's quite a bit of debate over whether or not absorbing magnesium through the skin is a viable option for supplementation. If you've done some research on the subject, you've likely read that magnesium is either best absorbed through the skin and/or that that's completely false and there's no reason to think that magnesium can be effectively absorbed in this way. As you might expect, the actual truth seems to fall somewhere between the two.

It's pretty well known that the skin is the largest organ of the body. In fact, it represents about 10 percent of the total body mass of an average person. Its main job is to act as a barrier between our internal environment and the outside world—covering us and protecting us from chemicals, allergens, germs, and the sun. This means that in many ways, the whole point of the skin is to *not* allow things to pass through it. To enter the bloodstream, magnesium would have to pass through layers and layers of tightly packed cells. Many scientists argue that hydrated magnesium ions, like those found in magnesium chloride, are way too big to pass through the biological membranes of our skin cells. This feels like bad news for those who are pro transdermal magnesium, but all hope is not lost! Magnesium could still potentially be absorbed by specific magnesium transporters—which we're still studying and gaining an understanding of—or through hair follicles or sweat glands, which provide ways to bypass the layers and layers of tightly packed cells in our skin.

There have been quite a few studies on whether or not transdermal magnesium is a viable way to get magnesium into the body. One study showed that magnesium ions can penetrate the outer layer of the skin by way of hair follicles and sweat glands, but it's still unclear if this occurs in amounts that would actually be therapeutic for humans because hair follicles and sweat glands only make up from 0.1 percent to 1 percent of the skin's surface. One source in particular that people in the pro transdermal magnesium camp tend to cite a lot says that transdermal application of magnesium can rectify a deficiency within four to six weeks compared to oral supplementation, which can take up to a year. Unfortunately, a full publication of that exact study can't be found, only an abstract from a conference is available, which suggests it wasn't actually published in a peer-reviewed journal.

A fair amount of the research published on transdermal magnesium is flawed in some way. For example, one study tested magnesium oil sprays and 20-minute magnesium foot soaks on nine patients. After 12 weeks there was a 59.7-percent increase in magnesium measured by analyzing hair follicles. This sounds great until you learn that the researchers did not state that they collected any information on blood serum magnesium concentration. Another group of researchers did actually measure blood concentrations of magnesium when they tested magnesium sulfate baths on 19 participants. All but three of them showed a rise in magnesium concentrations in blood plasma, and the researchers concluded that "prolonged soaking in Epsom salts increases blood magnesium concentrations." Interestingly, the patients who didn't have an increase in serum magnesium had larger increases in urine magnesium levels, which they also measured. This suggests that those patients already had optimal levels of magnesium in their body, so the excess magnesium was simply excreted by the kidneys. Unfortunately, this study was not published in a peer-reviewed journal but by the Epsom Salt Council, so take it with a grain of, well, *salt*.

If you're interested in learning more about the transdermal magnesium debate, check out an article published in the journal *Nutrients* titled "Myth or Reality—Transdermal Magnesium?" It's a great resource and really delves into the science, concluding: "Magnesium might be able to get into the lymphatic system beneath the dermis and enter the circulatory system, bypassing the regulation through the GI tract and hereby increasing serum magnesium. However, we cannot yet recommend the application of transdermal magnesium." I think this is a very fair and balanced conclusion.

The reality is that I could write pages and pages (and pages) on this topic. And while I don't want to say that it would be a total waste of time, it would be pretty boring and it would be missing the most important point, which is that despite the doubts about if and how magnesium can be absorbed through the skin, there are thousands of people using it this way. There are also thousands of health practitioners who have seen it work well for their patients, and they will keep recommending it, despite the lack of research and questions about the exact science.

Knowing all this, if you have a confirmed deficiency or if you're taking magnesium for a specific condition—like migraines or as part of a larger plan for managing diabetes—I suggest that you stick with oral supplementation. If you're experimenting with magnesium for general stress management or relaxation, experimenting with topical magnesium could be a good option for you. Keep in mind that it's thought that magnesium chloride is more effective than magnesium sulfate for actually raising magnesium levels in your blood. The effects of magnesium salt baths seem to be pleasant, relaxing, and pain relieving—but short-lived. Magnesium chloride is more easily assimilated and metabolized, and so less of it is needed for absorption. An added bonus of applying magnesium to the skin? You bypass the digestive system so there's no risk of giving yourself the runs if you take too much of the wrong form of magnesium.

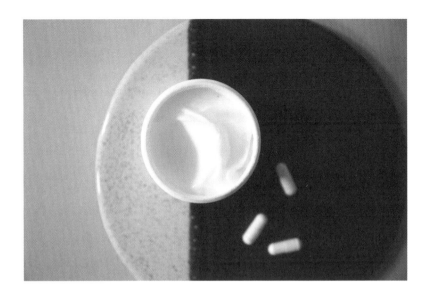

The debate over magnesium creams and sprays is an interesting one. Personally, when I use these creams and sprays on my feet before bed I sleep like a rock. I'd even compare it to taking NyQuil, minus the grogginess the next day. I have found that Epsom salt baths also do wonders for my post-workout soreness, for times when I'm stressed, or when my body is achy and in pain for any reason, like if I have the flu. I use them all the time, which probably won't come as a surprise seeing as I'm the author of this book, but I don't rely on them as my *only* source of magnesium intake.

## THE PROS AND CONS OF IV MAGNESIUM SUPPLEMENTS

Now that we've put the transdermal magnesium question to rest, we can move on to the debate over IV magnesium supplements, and really, IV supplements in general. To me, IV supplements feel extreme for a few reasons. They can be very expensive and there are always risks when needles are involved. This is also a good time to remind you that when it comes to alternative treatments and "out there" wellness practices, if it seems too good to be true, it probably is. Just like oral supplements, IV infusions aren't a magic bullet for better health. They're just one more tool we have at our disposal. In most situations, if you're not feeling your best, then you should try to identify areas of your everyday lifestyle—such as your sleep habits, exercise routine, nutrition protocols, and stress levels—that might need adjusting before you go looking for an external solution.

There are, however, a few reasons why I might consider an IV supplement. The first is pretty simple: if my doctor recommended it. Doctors might do this for migraines or to help reverse a clinically diagnosed deficiency more quickly. Another reason would be if a patient has IBS (irritable bowel syndrome) or leaky gut—or some other gut dysfunction—that prevented them from effectively absorbing minerals through their GI tract. As I mentioned before, I might also consider them if I was suffering from an illness like chronic fatigue or fibromyalgia, or even something like chronic insomnia—as IV supplements are a quick way to see if a nutrient might bring any relief.

That said, these infusions are expensive (it isn't easy to find one for less than $100) and they take about 30 minutes. I've had an IV of magnesium once or twice and let me tell you, I definitely felt the effect. I felt relaxed and sleepy almost immediately, and the feeling lasted for a few days. Pro tip: I would not recommend getting an IV of magnesium early in the day if you have a lot to do. I made this mistake and was so tired and relaxed I could barely function at work! In conclusion, the pros of IV infusions are that they're very bioavailable and customizable to the individual. The downsides are their price and potential risks. I'll leave it up to you and your doctor to decide what's best for your unique health *and* financial situation.

Understandably, you might be in a state of information overload. But don't stress! You can always just begin with a magnesium citrate supplement in capsule form or a simple Epsom salt bath—they are good options to start off with. Luckily, magnesium supplements at the recommended dosage are generally very safe and generally inexpensive, so you can test them out and adjust the brand and delivery method until you find one that works for you, your lifestyle, and your specific health goals.

# 7

# Taking Magnesium for the First Time

Now that you've chosen a magnesium supplement that is both high quality and right for your specific needs, the next step is to make sure you're well versed in safety and dosing. If you're nervous about taking magnesium, just remember that you're getting it through your diet every day already—and in pretty high amounts if your diet includes leafy greens, nuts, and seeds. To me, it's comforting to know that magnesium isn't a synthetic substance or even an herb that your body might not be used to processing. That being said, there's important information on dosing, safety, and medication interactions that you should know about before you take magnesium for the very first time.

When it comes to dosing magnesium, it's not all that simple. Before we go any further, I want to remind you again—even though I sound like a broken record—that you should always talk to your doctor before trying new supplements or making any drastic changes to your lifestyle routine, especially if you have a chronic health condition or are taking any medications. Without further ado, here are some important things to know about taking magnesium safely.

## YOUR GO-TO GUIDE TO DOSING MAGNESIUM

The recommended daily allowances (RDAs) for magnesium are 310 to 320 milligrams for adult women and 400 to 420 milligrams for adult men. Researchers think that the average person is only getting around 200 to 250 mg of magnesium through their food each day, so many of us need to supplement to get to the official RDA. Keep in mind that these official RDAs are just guidelines and don't necessarily account for all of the factors that can leave us depleted in magnesium. This explains why integrative and functional medicine experts will recommend taking 300 mg (or even as much as 500 mg a day if you have a deficiency) of magnesium daily in supplemental form on top of making an effort to eat magnesium-rich foods. It's not recommended that you take more than 350 mg of supplemental magnesium a day unless directed by a health care practitioner.

If you're taking one of the forms of magnesium known for causing digestive upset if you take too much, start with a low dose (around 150 mg a day) and then slowly increase your dose until you reach the RDA. Remember, the amount of magnesium you actually absorb depends on your current magnesium status, the health of your gut, and the form of magnesium you're taking. The National Institutes of Health (NIH) official dosage recommendations are:

- Infants–6 months: 30 milligrams
- 7–12 months: 75 milligrams
- 1–3 years: 80 milligrams
- 4–8 years: 130 milligrams
- 9–13 years: 240 milligrams
- 14–18 years: 410 milligrams for men; 360 milligrams for women
- 19–30 years: 400 milligrams for men; 310 milligrams for women
- Adults 31 years and older: 420 milligrams for men; 320 milligrams for women
- Pregnant women: 350–360 milligrams
- Women who are breastfeeding: 310–320 milligrams

You'll notice that the NIH recommends increasing your intake of magnesium by 30 to 50 milligrams per day during pregnancy. As it turns out, magnesium is important for maintaining nerve and muscle cell health, and it also helps regulate body temperature and protein synthesis, which are all very important during pregnancy. A randomized, controlled trial published in *Advanced Biomedical Research* in 2017 shows that maintaining optimal levels of magnesium during pregnancy is associated with better pregnancy outcomes. Specifically, that maintaining optimal levels of magnesium might help reduce the risk of the uterus contracting prematurely, decrease fetal growth restriction, and increase birth weight. Research has also shown that taking magnesium sulfate intravenously is associated with bone thinning in the fetus—which prompted the FDA to release a safety statement on the topic in 2013 titled "FDA Recommends Against Prolonged Use of Magnesium Sulfate to Stop Pre-term Labor Due to Bone Changes in Exposed Babies"—so the type of magnesium you supplement with during pregnancy matters. If you're pregnant, magnesium is something you can chat about with your OB/GYN if you haven't already!

## CAN YOU OVERDOSE ON MAGNESIUM?

Now for the question we've all been waiting for: Can you take too much magnesium? From everything I've surmised, it would be very challenging to overdose on magnesium-rich foods, but it is definitely possible to take too much magnesium in supplement form. The most common symptoms from taking too much magnesium are diarrhea and abdominal cramping, which I've mentioned quite a few times already. These symptoms are more common with magnesium carbonate, chloride, gluconate, and oxide than with other forms of magnesium. If you really take too much, you can experience hypotension, flushing, nausea, and vomiting. At even higher doses you can get severe hypermagnesemia, which is very uncommon but can lead to neuromuscular dysfunction, respiratory depression, and even coma. There have even been a few recorded cases of fatal hypermagnesemia (one in an elderly man and one in a young child). These deaths were linked to overdosing on magnesium-containing laxatives and antacids, which can contain more than 5,000 mg of magnesium. This risk is something we should all be aware of; but also keep in mind that you have to take an *enormous amount of magnesium* to put yourself at risk for a true magnesium overdose.

So who should be cautious about magnesium overdose, and who is more at risk for hypermagnesemia? If you have an issue with your kidneys—like impaired renal function or kidney failure—you'll want to talk to your doctor before taking magnesium and you will want to be extra cautious because, as we've learned, your kidneys work to regulate magnesium homeostasis in the body. Another reason to think twice about taking magnesium is if you have low blood pressure, because magnesium can lower it even further.

## WILL MAGNESIUM INTERACT WITH ANY OF YOUR MEDICATIONS?

There are several medications that magnesium can interact with. This isn't an exhaustive list, but some of the common ones are bisphosphonates, diuretics, and antibiotics. Bisphosphonates are drugs that are used to treat osteoporosis and magnesium can decrease their ability to be absorbed in the body. You *can* take both, but they should not be taken at the exact same time of day. The general recommendation is to leave at least two hours between taking magnesium and a bisphosphonate drug. Other medications such as diuretics and proton pump inhibitors can deplete your body of magnesium or interfere with the effectiveness of supplementing with oral magnesium, so you might actually need to supplement with higher doses of magnesium than the average person— or try alternate delivery methods. Also, antibiotics can interact with magnesium supplements. If you have to take antibiotics, you can either pause your magnesium supplementation until the round is over or you can talk to your doctor about the safest way to space them out.

## HOW LONG WILL MAGNESIUM TAKE TO WORK?

So now on to one of the most important questions that I am asked all the time: How long will it take to notice a difference when you start taking magnesium? That all depends on your personal biochemistry and also how and why you're taking magnesium in the first place. If you're getting an IV of magnesium, you might notice a difference before you've even finished the treatment (I know I did). If you're taking Epsom salt baths for something to help with sleep or anxiety, you might also notice immediate benefits. If you're taking oral magnesium supplements in search of better blood sugar balance or to help with another type of chronic condition, it would behoove you to take magnesium for at least two to three weeks before you make any final judgements, assuming you're not having any negative side effects like loose stools. And as I mentioned earlier, correcting a deficiency could take as long as a year. This might seem like a long time, but herbs and supplements are a gentler, whole-body approach to health issues, and therefore, they require a lot of time, consistency, and patience. Of course, you should make other lifestyle changes in addition to taking them.

So there you have it! You now have some important tools at your disposal to start taking advantage of magnesium in a way that is well informed—from the origins of Epsom salt baths and the amount of magnesium in our bones to how much it is recommended you take and which health conditions it might help to alleviate. In the next few chapters, I'll give you some inspiration for integrating magnesium into your kitchen and daily self-care routine.

# 8

# Magnesium in the Kitchen

This is where the real fun begins! It feels like every day someone discovers a new way to incorporate magnesium into a daily routine. To me, that's really exciting because taking a bunch of supplements every day can be a drag. It can also make you feel like a patient, ironic since the reason why many people turn to natural remedies is because they are disillusioned with pills, conventional health care, and the limited treatment options they feel they've been given.

As I've mentioned before, I always prefer to get my nutrients through food first, and only then do I turn to supplements. I also typically prefer supplements that can be incorporated into my day in a natural and seamless way. An example of this would be drinking lots of nettle tea (which I do religiously in the springtime) for allergies, instead of taking a capsule, or drinking some golden milk (a traditional Ayurvedic tonic made with turmeric) every night before bed instead of taking a turmeric supplement. Other good examples would be using CBD oil as a topical cream for jaw pain or taking your mushrooms for immunity in a delicious mushroom hot chocolate at the end of the day instead of in a capsule. Given the option, I will always choose a tincture or a powder. Luckily, there are many ways to use magnesium that don't involve a pill at all.

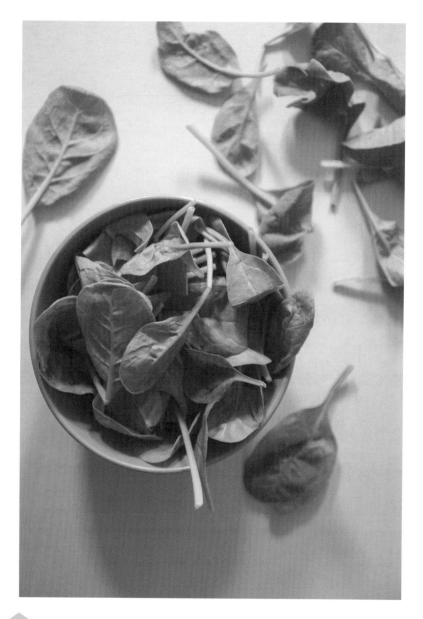

## GETTING BETTER ACQUAINTED WITH MAGNESIUM-RICH FOODS

On the following pages, you'll find a mix of recipes featuring foods that are high in magnesium and that feature supplemental magnesium either as a liquid or powder. Remember, magnesium is found in a wide variety of plant and animal foods, and some important ones are:

- Green leafy vegetables such as spinach, kale, collard greens, turnip greens, and mustard greens
- Legumes such as black beans and lentils
- Fruits such as figs, avocados, and bananas
- Nuts and seeds, especially pumpkin seeds, squash seeds, sesame seeds, almonds, and cashews
- Whole grains
- Yogurt and kefir
- Fatty fish such as salmon, mackerel, halibut, and tuna
- Dark chocolate

### Soaking and Sprouting Nuts and Seeds

Did you know that soaking and sprouting nuts, seeds, and grains can make the magnesium they contain more bioavailable to your body? It's true. These processes can also make these foods easier for you to digest and remove some of their harmful enzymes and ingredients such as phytic acid, which can interfere with nutrient absorption and be harmful to your gut. Sprouting your own foods can be time intensive, but luckily, a lot of stores sell presprouted products. Soaking nuts and seeds is easy, just soak them overnight in warm water and salt—like in the Raspberry Buckwheat Overnight Oats recipe (see page 116). You can also check out the recipe for Homemade Pumpkin Seed Milk (see page 103) to understand what soaking actually entails. You can use that pumpkin seed milk recipe to make a variety of nut and seed milks. This method is a great way to make sure you're getting as much magnesium from them as possible, make them easier to digest, and avoid the added sugars, gums, and emulsifiers (like carrageenan) found in many store-bought nut and seed milks.

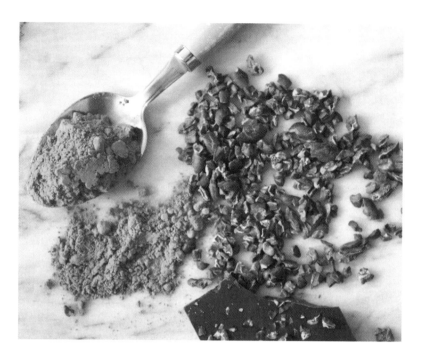

## MY OVERALL FOOD PHILOSOPHY: WHY IT'S
## GOOD NEWS FOR YOUR MAGNESIUM INTAKE

The recipes I've included in this book are largely plant based. The few exceptions are ghee, a form of clarified butter that I love to incorporate into recipes, and a little bit of kefir, which you can always substitute for nondairy coconut or almond milk kefir. These nondairy products, however, don't add the tangy tartness I prefer in some dishes such as Mango Cream Chia Pudding (see page 120). You might notice that I've left grains out of these recipes almost entirely. That is because the magnesium content of certain grains and cereals is typically high because the grains and cereals have been fortified (meaning magnesium has been added to them when it wasn't there before). Then there are also some that are enriched, which is different from fortified. Enriching foods is when companies add vitamins and minerals back into a food that were lost during processing. I'm not a fan of processed, fortified, or enriched foods; I'm more interested in real, whole foods that come straight from Mother Nature with their magnesium intact.

You'll also notice that almost nothing in these recipes is cooked. Uncooked foods preserve the magnesium content more than cooked foods. Keep in mind that the foods we're eating today don't have the same amount of magnesium as they once did because of soil depletion. For this reason, if you think you have a magnesium deficiency (or you have confirmed it through one of the tests I mentioned earlier), then you'll probably want to focus your energies on both magnesium supplements *and* magnesium-rich foods and drinks. These recipes highlight magnesium, but they're also full of ingredients that are healthy for a ton of reasons. Their magnesium content is just an added bonus.

Are you ready to get started? Here are 15 recipes to help you up your magnesium intake through delicious smoothies, snacks, and desserts. Keep in mind that these recipes—and the self-care recipes in Chapter 9—were designed for adults and that it's always important to talk to a health care provider before adding anything to your wellness regime.

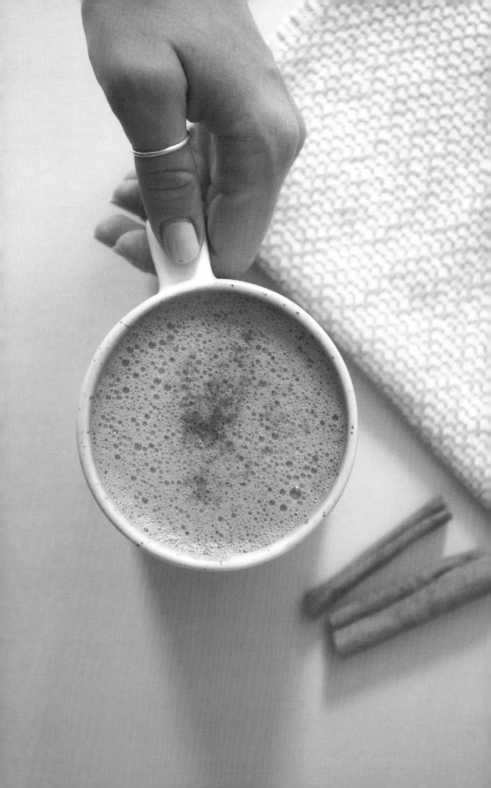

# Pumpkin Spice Latte

*If only I could transport myself back to high school when I didn't know how unhealthy pumpkin spiced lattes were. Because once you know, you can never forget. The good news is that you can usually create a healthy version of an unhealthy food (with a little creativity, of course). This pumpkin spice latte is made with rooibos tea and canned pumpkin with no sugar added. I recommend quadrupling the pumpkin mixture and then storing it in the fridge so you can enjoy these lattes for a few days in a row. To add some sweetness you'll use molasses, which is extra credit because it's also high in magnesium—one tablespoon typically contains about 40 mg of my favorite mineral.*

**MAKES 1 SERVING**

## Ingredients

1 cup nondairy milk (I like almond milk)

1 cup hot water

1 rooibos tea bag (I like the Numi Organic Tea, Rooibos Chai for this recipe)

2 tablespoons pumpkin purée

½ teaspoon ground ginger

1 teaspoon molasses

½ teaspoon cinnamon

¼ teaspoon nutmeg

## Method

1. Add milk and water to a small saucepan and heat on medium until you see steam rising from the pan. Turn heat to low and add tea bag, cover, and let steep for 5 minutes.
2. Add pumpkin, ginger, cinnamon, and molasses and stir until they're fully incorporated.
3. Transfer to a blender and blend on high until there is plenty of froth, then pour into your favorite mug, sprinkle with a bit of nutmeg, and enjoy immediately.

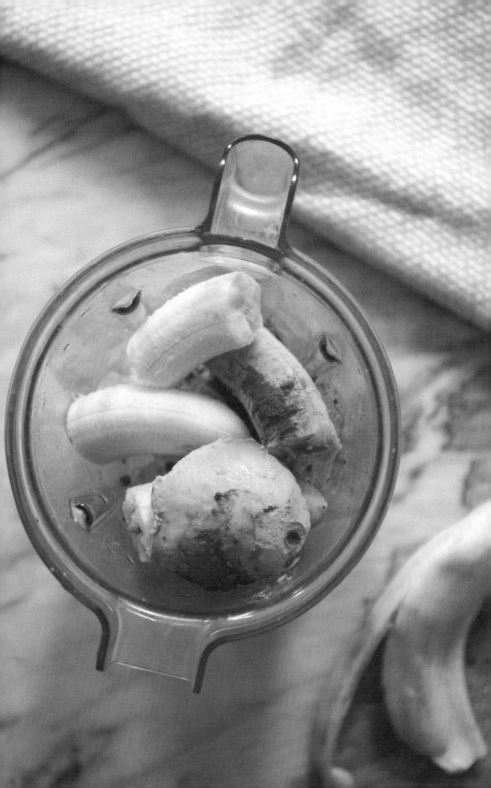

# Avocado Mocha Smoothie

Thank goodness chocolate has high amounts of magnesium, *are words I uttered to myself quite a few times while developing recipes for this book. Chocolate is one of the most versatile foods out there and is, of course, a fan favorite. This smoothie is low in sugar and contains a shot of espresso (I'm obsessed with my Nespresso Espresso machine), making it perfect for breakfast or for that notorious 3 p.m. slump. It's reminiscent of my favorite sugar-filled, barista-made drink—but without the massive amounts of added sugar, dairy, massive amounts of caffeine, and hefty price tag. It features cacao powder, which typically offers about 40 mg of magnesium per tablespoon.*

## MAKES 1 SERVING

### Ingredients

1 large frozen banana

½ frozen avocado

1 teaspoon cacao powder

½ teaspoon alcohol-free vanilla
   extract

1 cup nondairy milk of choice
   (I like using lightly sweetened
   [less than 7 grams of sugar]
   vanilla hemp milk with this one)

20 grams (about 2 scoops)
   unflavored collagen powder

Single shot of espresso or 2
   ounces of extra strong coffee

1 teaspoon cacao nibs

### Method

1. Add frozen banana, avocado, cacao powder, vanilla, milk, and collagen powder to a high-speed blender. Blend until fully incorporated.
2. Pour espresso shot on top and pulse for 2 seconds to get that fun Frappuccino effect. Top with cacao nibs for a nice crunch.

# Avocado Pistachio Ice Cream

*There aren't many things in life better than cozying up in bed to watch a movie with a bowl of ice cream—and my absolute favorite flavor is pistachio. This recipe was designed to fulfill a craving for this cold treat in a way that's actually good news for your health. This ice cream is dairy free and has significantly less sugar than store-bought ice cream. And, of course, it's full of magnesium from the pistachios, which contain about 140 mg of magnesium per cup.*

**MAKES 4 SERVINGS**

## Ingredients

1 tablespoon coconut oil

1 cup pistachios, shelled

½ cup honey

½ teaspoon cardamom

½ teaspoon almond extract

½ teaspoon vanilla extract

½ teaspoon salt

1 cup almond milk

3 ripe avocados, frozen

## Method

1. Add coconut oil to a medium sauté pan and bring to medium heat. Add pistachios, honey, cardamom, almond extract, vanilla extract, and salt. Cook until pistachios start browning ever so slightly and you can smell their aroma. Turn off heat and allow to cool slightly, around 5 minutes. Add almond milk and stir frequently until the color of the milk is even throughout.
2. Allow to cool completely.
3. Transfer contents of pan into a blender, add avocados, and blend until it resembles soft serve ice cream. Pour into a sheet pan, cover with aluminum foil or plastic wrap, and put in the freezer for at least 2 hours. When you're ready to enjoy, just scoop right out of the pan with an ice cream scooper or large metal spoon.

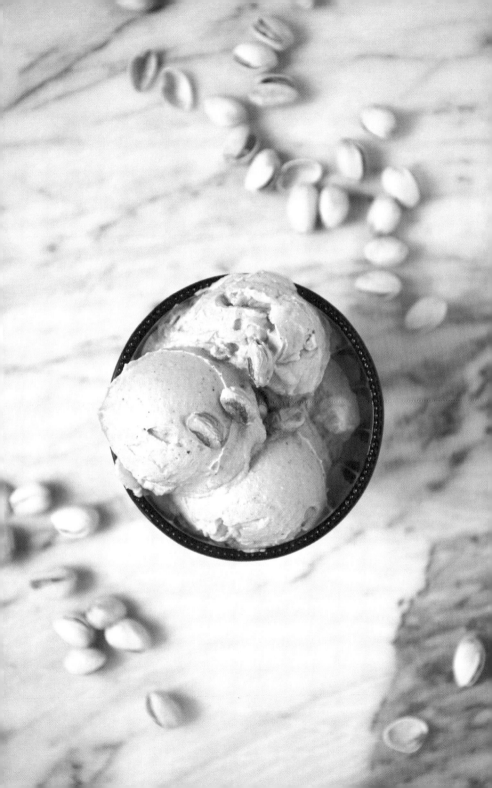

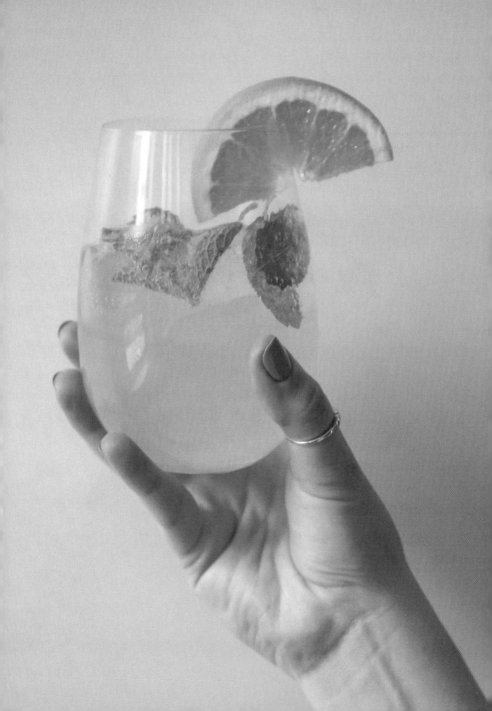

# Magnesium Spritz

*Like most millennials these days, I'm obsessed with the Aperol Spritz. That said, I try to minimize my alcohol intake as much as possible because even one drink seems to zap my energy levels the next day. Because of this, I've gotten into making low-sugar mocktails that satisfy my desire to have something colorful and delicious. I drink it out of a tall glass with a fun straw (plastic free and reusable, of course). This "spritz" is made with orange, bitters, soda water, and my favorite orange-flavored magnesium drink. Pro tip: If you're adding the orange zest, make sure to buy an organic orange, and wash and rinse the rind thoroughly.*

## MAKES 2 SERVINGS

### Ingredients

1 orange, juiced

5 shakes grapefruit or orange bitters

16 ounces sparkling water

1 dose (typically around 350 mg) of powdered magnesium (I like Natural Vitality, Natural Calm, Orange Flavor; or if you want to add some sweetness, try Thorne's Magnesium Bisglycinate powder, which is sweetened with monk fruit concentrate)

Pinch of orange zest

### Method

1. Pick out your two favorite wine glasses and fill them with ice.
2. Squeeze the juice out of ½ of the orange into each glass.
3. Add grapefruit bitters, sparkling water, magnesium, and orange zest.
4. Stir until all ingredients are fully incorporated and enjoy chilled! If you're feeling fancy, top with an orange slice.

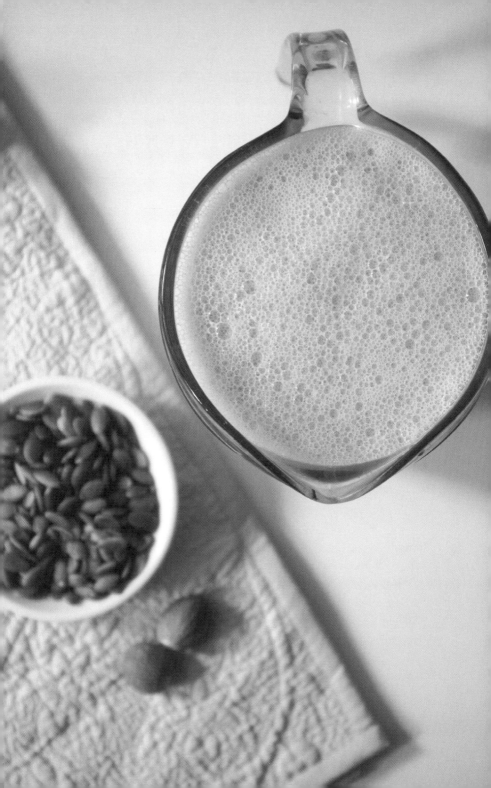

# Homemade Pumpkin Seed Milk

*A great way to get a daily dose of magnesium is by making your own homemade nut or seed milk. Pumpkin seeds are one of my favorite foods in the world and they just so happen to be very high in magnesium—providing about 150 mg of magnesium per cup. You can use any nut or seed in this recipe. Other nuts high in magnesium include almonds, cashews, and hemp seeds. With this simple recipe, you can avoid the added sugars, gums, and fillers found in many store-bought nut milks.*

**MAKES 4 SERVINGS**

### Ingredients

1 cup pumpkin seeds

1 teaspoon salt

4 cups warm water

1 large date

½ teaspoon nutmeg

1 teaspoon vanilla extract
   (alcohol-free)

### Method

1. Place pumpkin seeds, salt, and water into a large mason jar and soak overnight on your kitchen counter (do not refrigerate).
2. The next day, strain the pumpkin seeds and rinse them gently. Transfer seeds to a blender and add 4 cups of fresh water, the date, nutmeg, and vanilla.
3. Blend on high until the milk is clump free and nice and frothy.
4. Store in a mason jar with a water-tight lid for up to 4 days, just remember to shake well before enjoying.

# Blood-Sugar-Balancing Cinnamon Bites

*This is my go-to recipe for those stress-induced sugar cravings. These bites are completely sugar free and chock-full of healthy fats and protein, which are great for calming cravings, plus magnesium-rich ingredients such as cashews, chia seeds, and cacao. To top things off, this recipe calls for a hefty dose of cinnamon, an ingredient that has blood sugar-stabilizing properties. In one study, volunteers who ate 1 to 6 grams of cinnamon for 40 days lowered their blood sugar levels by 24 percent.*

**MAKES 5 SERVINGS**

### Ingredients

½ teaspoon unsweetened vanilla extract

2 tablespoons chia seeds

1 cup organic oats

⅓ cup cashew butter or nut butter of your choice

1 tablespoon coconut oil

2 teaspoons cinnamon

⅛ teaspoon Himalayan pink sea salt

¼ teaspoon ground ginger

¼ cup goji berries (optional)

### Method

1. Add nut butter, vanilla extract, cinnamon, ginger, salt, oats, and coconut oil to a food processor and blend until all ingredients are fully incorporated.
2. Transfer to a bowl and fold in chia seeds. Refrigerate for 45 minutes, then shape into tablespoon-sized balls. Sprinkle with a few additional chia seeds or goji berries.

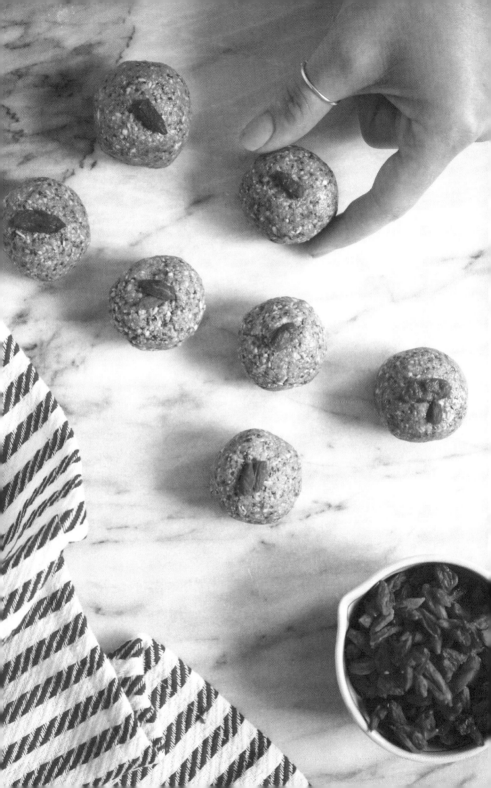

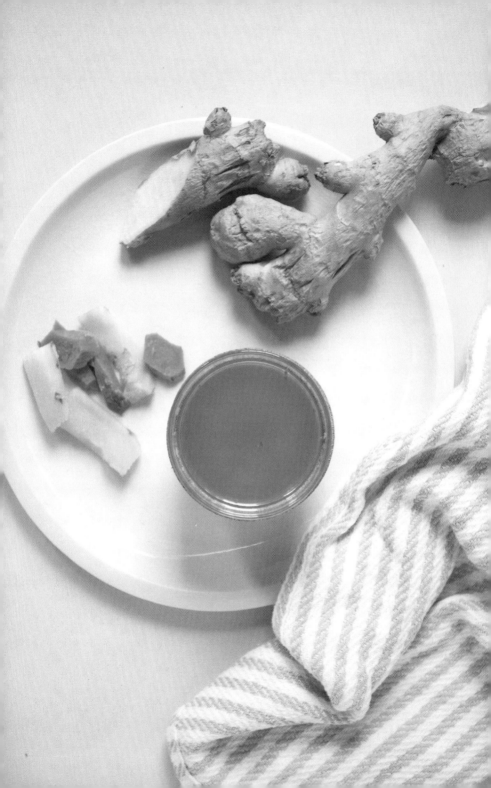

# P.M. Digestion-Support Tonic

*Warning! This one makes me feel like an ancient healer brewing up a digestive potion in my laboratory. I enjoy it at the end of a long day or after a meal out with friends when my belly needs a little TLC. Ginger and fennel are digestive system superstars, and a little bit of healthy fat can help coat and soothe the digestive tract. The honey is optional— because it's not a great idea to consume sugar before you go to bed—but it adds some sweetness in case this one is a little too strong for you on its own.*

**MAKES 2 SERVINGS**

### Ingredients

1 clove fresh gingerroot, chopped finely

1 clove fresh turmeric root, chopped finely

1 teaspoon fennel seeds, pulverized or ground

1 teaspoon honey (optional)

1 teaspoon ghee or olive oil

### Method

1. Heat water on stove in a small saucepan until boiling. Turn heat to low and add ginger, turmeric, and fennel seeds. Cover and let it sit about 15 minutes (longer if you're not afraid of a little extra spice).
2. Pour tonic through a strainer into a cup, add honey, if using, and ghee and stir. Enjoy after dinner, before bed, or whenever you're struggling with bloating or indigestion.

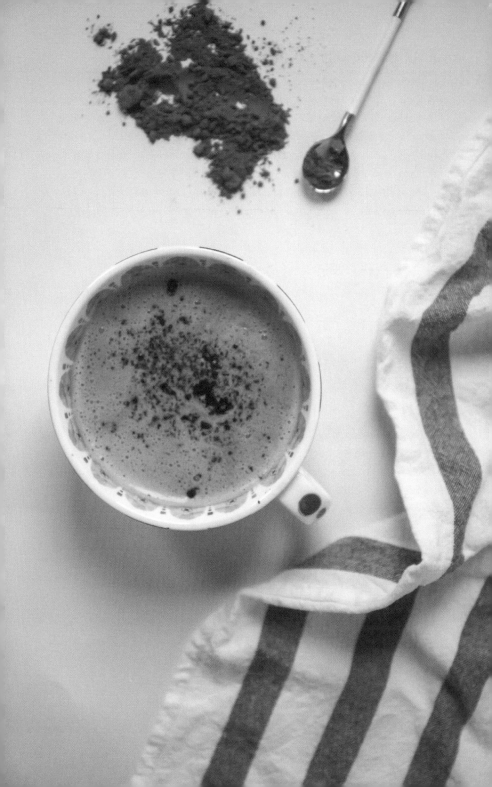

# Beet Hazelnut Latte

*Beets have a very impressive nutritional profile, making them a great choice for getting some essential vitamins and minerals—especially magnesium and iron. This is the perfect drink when I'm feeling drained, especially if my fatigue is menstrual-cycle related. It's also convenient: Many health experts suggest avoiding caffeine during that time of the month, because it might exacerbate whatever symptoms you're already feeling. Sprinkle a little bit of cacao powder to top off this beet latte and it becomes an amazing (caffeine-free) afternoon drink that tastes ever-so-slightly like Nutella.*

**MAKES 1 SERVING**

### Ingredients

1 fresh beet or 2 to 3 ounces of fresh beet juice

⅛ teaspoon almond extract

1 cup hazelnut milk (I'm obsessed with Elmhurst's hazelnut milk)

¼ teaspoon cacao powder, plus more for sprinkling

### Method

1. Cut off stems of beet and chop beet in half; add each half to a juicer, one at a time, and collect beet juice. It should make about 3 ounces of beet juice. Pour into the bottom of a mug (or clear glass if you have one; this drink is beautiful!).
2. Heat hazelnut milk in a small saucepan on low heat on the stove until you see steam rising from the pan. Add cacao powder and almond extract and stir until fully incorporated.
3. Pour milk over beet juice and sprinkle with cacao powder. Enjoy!

# Electrolyte Recovery Drink

*When you sweat, you lose a lot of electrolytes—including sodium, potassium, and magnesium. Ironically, the better shape you're in the more you sweat, according to research, like a study published in the journal* PLOS ONE *titled "Long Distance Runners Present Upregulated Sweating Responses than Sedentary Counterparts." This recovery drink is for those workout days when you feel spent and it seems like you've sweat out a few pounds of water at least. This drink is made from coconut water and Himalayan pink sea salt, which can help your body replenish the large amounts of potassium and salt that you have sweat out. You can add any powdered magnesium to this one, but I recommend Mineral$_2$O powder by Pure Encapsulations. It features the normal minerals such as sodium, potassium, and chloride, and it also contains a trace mineral complex that contains over 72 naturally occurring trace minerals found in seawater.*

**MAKES 1 SERVING**

## Ingredients:

1 cup cold filtered water

⅛ teaspoon Himalayan pink sea salt

1 scoop (around 1.8 g) of Pure Encapsulations Mineral$_2$O powder

1 cup coconut water (I like Harmless Harvest coconut water)

1 fresh lemon, juiced

## Method

1. Fill a pint mason jar ¼ full with pink sea salt crystals and the remaining ¾ full with filtered water. Put the lid on and shake, then leave the jar on the counter overnight (there should still be some undissolved salt in the bottom of the mason jar). This is called sole water and you can keep the solution on your kitchen counter for future use.

2. Take out one teaspoon of sole water and add to a large glass, then add mineral powder, coconut water, and 1 cup cold filtered water and stir. Add the lemon juice, stir again, and then drink it down!

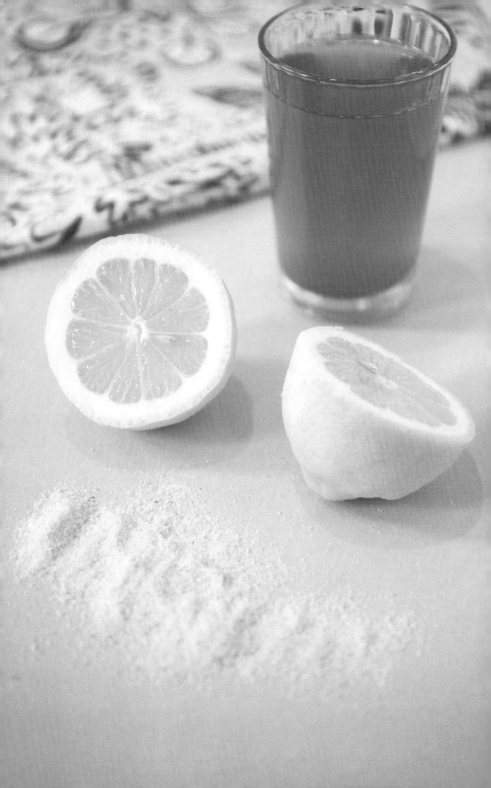

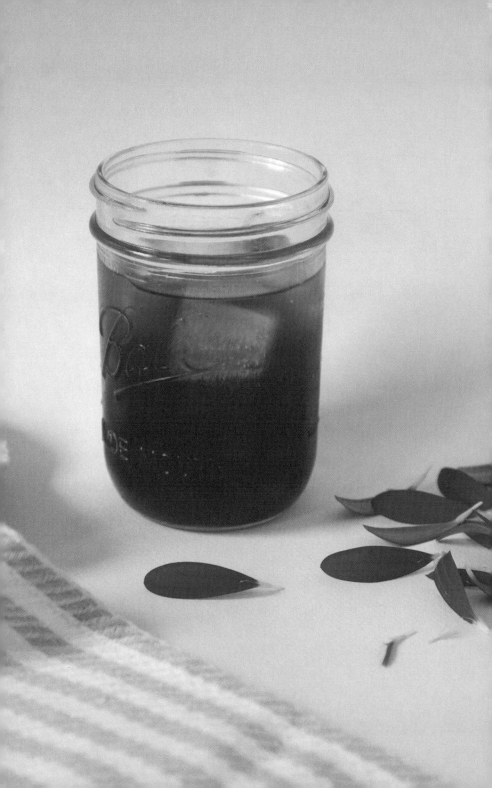

# Hibiscus Beauty Water

*I love the concept of beauty from the inside out. I have found, firsthand, that eating a healthy diet, taking time for self-care, and being mindful make me feel more attractive. This antioxidant- and mineral-rich beauty water is meant to cleanse your insides and to fight the free radicals that can lead to premature aging and wrinkles. This drink features hibiscus (rich in antioxidants that are especially beneficial to the skin) and liquid magnesium. I prefer this one over ice.*

**MAKES 2 SERVINGS**

## Ingredients

2 bags hibiscus tea (I like Gaia Herbs' Organic Hibiscus Tea)

1 tablespoon pomegranate powder (I like Navitas Naturals Certified Organic Pomegranate Powder)

1 dose unflavored liquid magnesium (if you're looking to splurge, use Sakara Life's Beauty Water Concentrate; it contains magnesium, chloride, trace minerals, and rose; the exact dose amount will depend on the brand you choose)

## Method

1. Fill medium saucepan with 2 cups of water on high heat. Once simmering, add hibiscus tea bags, turn off the heat, and then leave covered while it cools.
2. To make beauty water, take 1 cup of hibiscus tea and pour over ice water. You can store the other cup of tea in the fridge in a mason jar to use later. Add pomegranate powder and liquid magnesium to iced hibiscus tea and stir thoroughly. Enjoy!

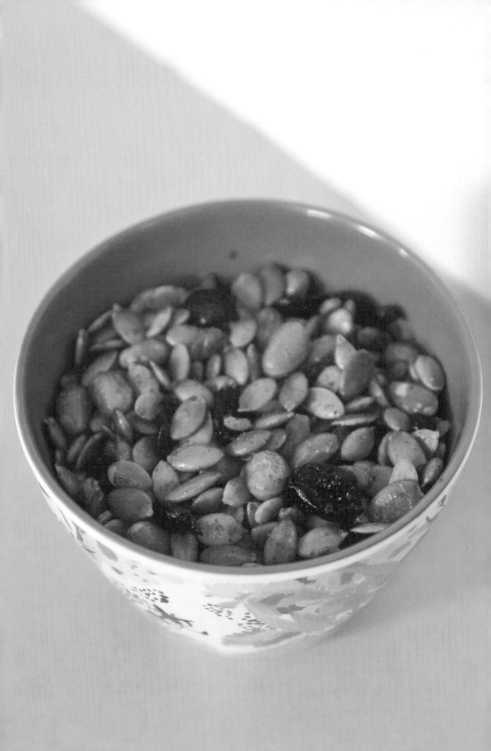

# Nut-Free Trail Mix

*Nuts are a great source of magnesium, but they can also be hard to digest for some people. In fact, I stopped eating nuts for a few months and I felt like my digestion really improved. Since then, I always look for go-to snacks that aren't a handful of cashews, a spoonful of nut butter, or a granola bar that inevitably features almonds or peanuts. This nut-free trail mix is a great go-to snack, plus it's easy to make on a sheet pan and embodies that irresistible mix of salty and sweet. Edamame is high in magnesium, and so are pumpkin seeds.*

**MAKES 2 SERVINGS**

### Ingredients

1 cup shelled edamame (defrosted or raw)

1 cup pumpkin seeds

1 tablespoon Madagascar vanilla bean ghee

1 teaspoon cinnamon

2 pinches Himalayan pink sea salt

½ teaspoon organic brown coconut sugar

½ cup dried cranberries (no sugar added)

### Method

1. Preheat oven to 350°F and line a sheet pan with parchment paper or aluminum foil.
2. In a large bowl, toss edamame and pumpkin seeds in ghee, cinnamon, salt, and coconut sugar.
3. Spread the mixture on the baking pan and bake for 10 minutes or until edamame looks nice and toasted and you can smell the pumpkin seeds wafting from the oven. Add cranberries and bake 5 to 7 more minutes.
4. Remove from oven and allow to cool a few minutes before enjoying.

# Raspberry Buckwheat Overnight Oats

*When I'm looking to up my magnesium intake and to get healthier in general, overnight oats and chia puddings are great recipes that I love to have in my arsenal. The best part about them is that they require almost no actual work; it's simply a matter of combining ingredients and letting them sit overnight. Buckwheat is one of my favorite foods in the world. It has such a strong nutty flavor that, in this recipe, is balanced out nicely by the mild sweetness of raspberries.*

**MAKES 1 SERVING**

## Ingredients

¼ cup old-fashioned, gluten-free rolled oats

¼ cup buckwheat groats

½ cup fresh raspberries

¾ cup nondairy milk of choice (I like Oatly! for this recipe)

1 tablespoon chopped walnuts or nuts of choice for topping

1 teaspoon honey for topping

## Method

1. Soak oats and groats overnight in warm water and salt. The next day, drain and rinse.
2. Add oats, groats, and all other ingredients to a mason jar; I like to layer the raspberries throughout and then top with a few raspberries, some walnuts, and a tiny drizzle of honey.
3. Allow mixture to sit overnight or at least 8 hours.
4. In the morning, simply grab and go. Just make sure you have a spoon!

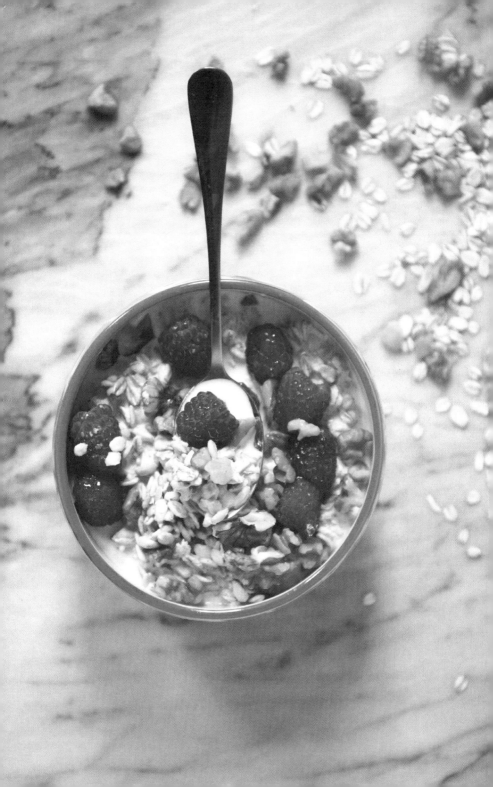

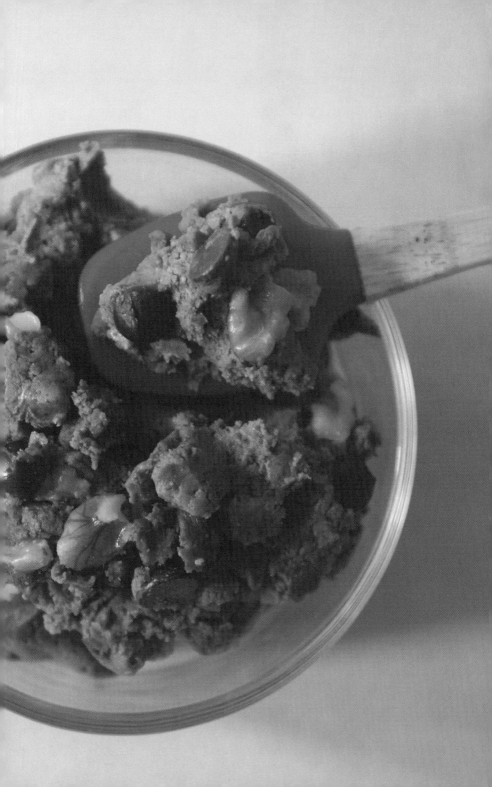

# Black Bean Brownie Batter

*Black beans are high in magnesium and one of the best ways to take advantage of this is to turn them into a homemade cookie dough or a brownie batter. This recipe is very low in sugar and the beans are high in fiber, so it makes for a pretty perfect afternoon snack. Heads up: You'll need a food processor for this one!*

**MAKES 2 SERVINGS**

## Ingredients

One (15-ounce) can of black beans, drained and rinsed

1½ teaspoons cacao powder

1 cup cashew butter

½ teaspoon pure vanilla extract

2 large dates or ¼ tablespoon date syrup (no sugar added)

⅓ cup dark chocolate chips

¼ teaspoon sea salt

½ cup chopped walnuts

## Method

1. Add black beans, cacao powder, cashew butter, and vanilla to a food processor and blend until creamy and all ingredients are fully dispersed.
2. Remove batter from food processor using a spatula and transfer to a large mixing bowl. Fold in chocolate chips, sea salt, and walnuts. Cover and refrigerate for 2 hours.
3. Remove dough from fridge and you can either transfer to a glass dish to store in the fridge or roll into bite-sized cookie dough bites.

# Mango Cream Chia Pudding

*Chia puddings and overnight oats are my go-tos for lazy days. This recipe is extra decadent. Sometimes, if I forget to bring it with me to work in the morning, I'll eat it for dessert in the evening. It's the perfect combo of tart, tangy, creamy, and not too sweet. Top with a few slices of mango and coconut flakes for a chia pudding that makes you feel like you're on vacation.*

**MAKES 1 SERVING**

### Ingredients

1 cup frozen mango

½ teaspoon ground ginger

1 cup organic kefir (I like Green Valley Organics)

2 tablespoons chia seeds

1 tablespoon organic coconut flakes

### Method

1. Add mango, ginger, and kefir to a blender and blend on high until fully mixed. Set aside.
2. In a medium-sized mason jar, add the chia seeds. Pour mixture from blender over chia seeds and stir. Close mason jar and shake before putting it into the fridge. A couple of hours later, shake again. Then let chia pudding sit overnight and sprinkle with coconut flakes before eating.

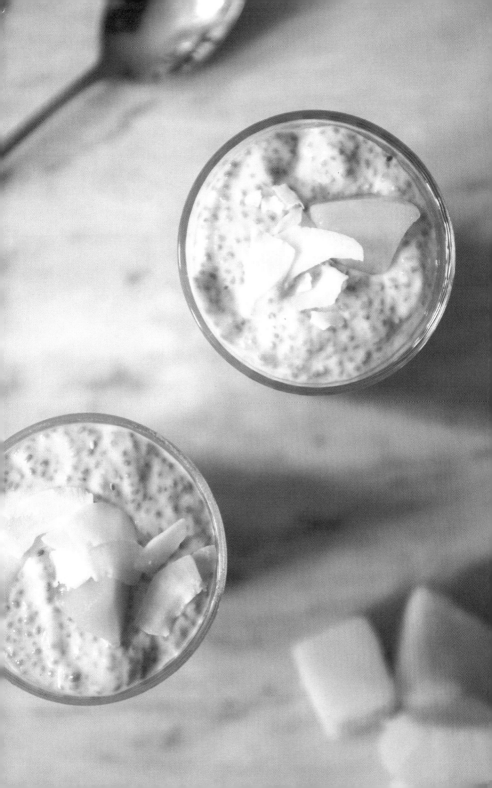

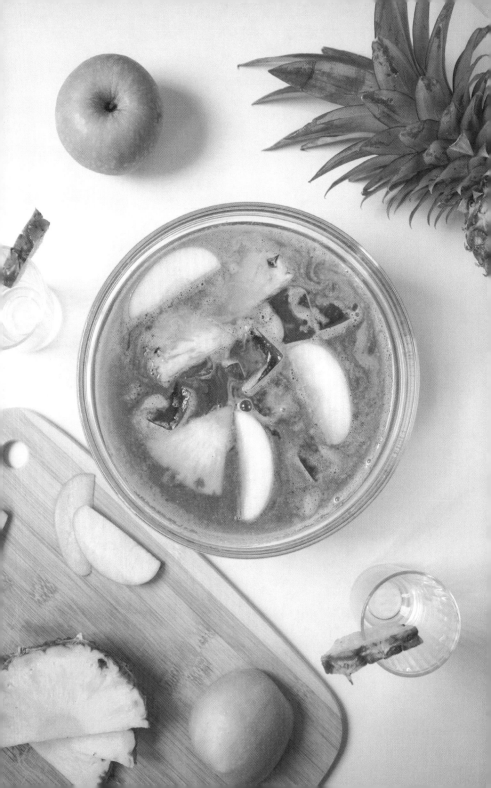

# Green Juice Punch

*If you want to shock (and then delight!) all your friends at your next party, this recipe is for you. Alcohol can deplete your body of magnesium, which is no good! If you have a healthy relationship with alcohol and want to try to replenish your body with essential vitamins, minerals, and antioxidants, then try combining your cocktail with a green juice. You can make juice yourself or you can pick up a green juice from your favorite juice bar. Simply combine it with your favorite vodka, add some ice and cold water, and voila! Make this one in a punch bowl or the biggest pitcher you have.*

**MAKES 8 SERVINGS**

### Ingredients

24 ounces green juice (you can use store-bought or juice kale, lemon, ginger, and green apple at home)

2 cups pineapple juice

1 cup cold water

2 cups ice

8 ounces (about 1 cup) of your favorite distilled vodka

½ green apple, sliced thinly for garnish

### Method

1. Combine all ingredients except for the vodka and apples in a punch bowl. Add vodka to taste.
2. Toss the apples in the bowl for a fun addition.

# 9

# Magnesium-Inspired Self-Care

Let the relaxation begin! The recipes on the following pages are meant to help you take advantage of the many beneficial properties of magnesium. They also encourage you to take some time for yourself. Luckily, transdermal magnesium is super versatile, and you have a lot of different creams and oils to choose from. Full disclosure, I have embedded a hidden agenda into this chapter, which is to help you reduce your use of both prescription drugs and over-the-counter medicines.

## REDUCING YOUR USE OF OTC MEDICATIONS WITH MAGNESIUM

We all know about the many side effects of common prescription medications, including painkillers, psychiatric medications, and amphetamines. Lesser known, though, are the many side effects of common over-the-counter drugs. When you really get into the nitty-gritty details, you might be shocked: The long-term use of anticholinergic drugs (this includes Benadryl and some other common medications) has been linked to an increased risk of developing dementia. Stomach bleeds from NSAIDs (nonsteroidal anti-inflammatory drugs) such as

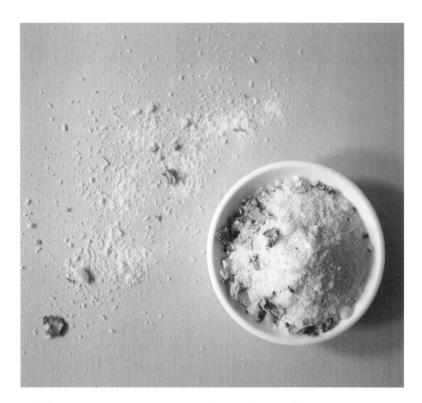

Advil are a very common reason why people visit the emergency room. In fact, around 103,000 hospitalizations and 16,500 deaths every year can be attributed to long-term NSAID use. Medications for acid reflux have been linked to severe nutrient deficiencies, and cold and cough medicines can interact with any number of other medications and are dangerous when mixed with alcohol.

I'm not trying to scare you; my point is that while you might not need a prescription to buy a bottle of Advil, it's not 100 percent safe, either. You should be aware of the risks of over-the-counter remedies in your medicine cabinet, especially if you're using them regularly. My goal with these recipes is not to convince you that all over-the-counter and prescription medications are useless or that you should avoid them at all costs, but, rather, I would like you to consider that in many situations a natural remedy can be tried first. Luckily, magnesium is an amazing natural ingredient for daily aches and pains and any number of health woes. For me, an Epsom salt bath or temple massage often acts as a substitute for over-the-counter pain relievers. I'll leave it up to you to decide what might work for you.

## DOSING TRANSDERMAL MAGNESIUM AND EPSOM SALTS

So how do you dose Epsom salts, magnesium oil, and other topical products? Typically, I recommend you use 1 to 2 cups of Epsom salts or magnesium chloride flakes per bath. This seems like a lot—now you know why the bags they sell them in are so big!—but don't skimp on the amount or you won't get the full beneficial results. Thankfully, Epsom salts are very reasonably priced so you don't have to stress too much about using them liberally.

As for dosing magnesium creams and oils, the rule of thumb is to just follow the directions on the label of whatever products you're using. Most of the time it will be about four sprays of magnesium oil and ¼ to 1 teaspoon at most of the gels, lotions, and creams. The good news is that the most common symptom of taking too much magnesium—diarrhea— usually isn't a factor with transdermal magnesium.

One more thing before diving into the recipes: Many of the bath recipes here incorporate essential oils. However, using them is not as simple as just dropping some directly into the bath water. It's always a good idea to dilute essential oils in a carrier oil before adding them to the bath, as they can be very potent and some can even burn the skin if undiluted. A good rule of thumb is to add 3 to 10 drops of essential oils to one tablespoon of a carrier oil such as coconut, jojoba, olive, apricot, or sweet almond before you add them to the bath. You can find these carrier oils next to the essential oils in most health food stores or you can get them online. *Warning:* Make sure to scrub the tub after your bath because the oil can remain and make your bathtub dangerously slippery.

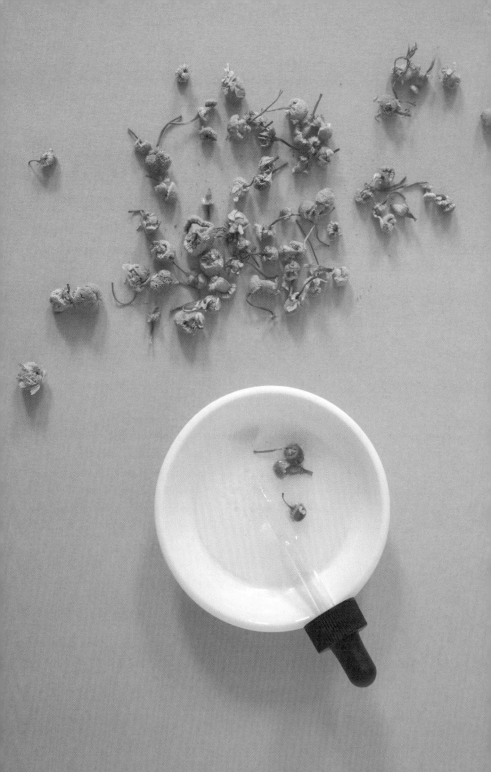

# Chamomile Body Oil

*What's the most relaxing thing in the universe? I'd have to say getting out of the shower after a long day and lathering myself, head to toe, in an amazing-smelling body oil. Adding chamomile and magnesium oil to the mix brings this ritual to a whole new level. An ounce of this oil (¼ of the final mixture) will contain about 100 mg of magnesium chloride. You can make it and keep it in a 4-ounce, colored glass spray bottle.*

**MAKES 1 TREATMENT**

## Ingredients

400 mg magnesium in a topical magnesium oil spray (I like Life-flo Pure Magnesium Oil)

4 droppersful (about 2,400 mg) chamomile liquid extract

2 ounces carrier oil of your choice (I like apricot oil for this remedy)

## Method

1. Combine the magnesium oil and chamomile extract in a 4-ounce, colored glass spray bottle. Fill to the top with carrier oil.
2. To use body oil, shake bottle thoroughly first, and massage oil into your feet, legs, arms, and the back of your neck before bed. You might notice that this leaves a little bit of white residue on your skin—this is just excess salt and can be easily wiped off in the shower or with a washcloth.

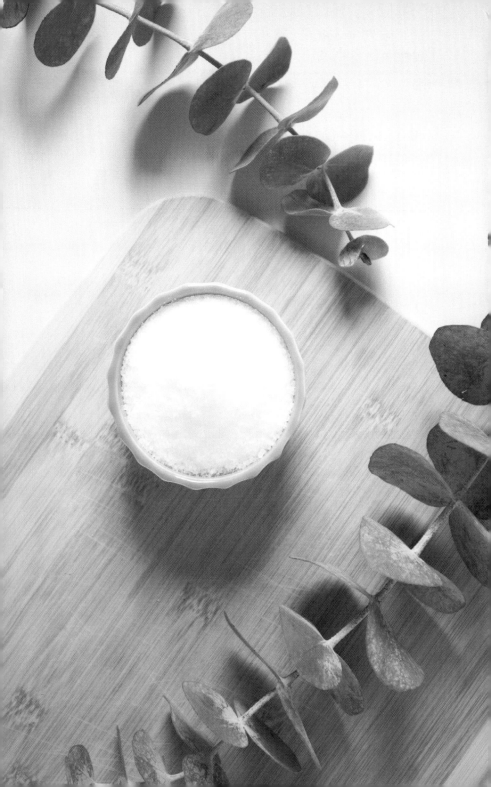

# End-of-Day Foot Soak

*I've been living in New York City for years, but it still surprises me how hard it is on my feet. At the end of the day, they just feel . . . sad. Whether we're standing all day, walking long distances, or just can't give up our stilettos, we don't appreciate all our feet do for us nearly enough. It's time to give them some TLC! I have a friend who is obsessed with foot health (yes, really). On top of this luxurious foot soak, she recommends regularly switching up your shoes, investing in arch supports if you need them, and using a lacrosse or tennis ball to massage your feet at the end of the day (or even better, while you're waiting on the water to heat up for this foot soak).*

**MAKES 1 TREATMENT**

### Ingredients

1 cup magnesium sulfate salts or magnesium chloride salts

3 drops eucalyptus essential oil

3 drops neroli essential oil

1 tablespoon of carrier oil

### Method

1. Heat some water on the stove or, if it gets hot enough, straight from the tap into a footbath or large container. You can also bring a chair to the side of your bathtub and dangle your feet right into the tub.
2. Add magnesium salts and essential oil along with carrier oil.
3. Stir with a wooden spoon or your hand until the salts are fully dissolved.
4. Soak feet for 15 to 20 minutes, adding more hot water as needed.

# CBD-MG Neck Rub

*I don't know about you, but my neck is* always sore. *Whether it's from writing, traveling, working out, or participating in any number of random activities (I'm looking at you, beach volleyball), my neck always seems to take a hit. I also, admittedly, hold a lot of my stress and tension in my upper shoulders, neck, and jaw. If this sounds like you, it's time to get proactive about soothing and relaxing those muscles. Once I discovered this epic combo of magnesium and CBD oil, I started using it every single night before bed and sometimes in the morning as well. It's been a big help!*

**MAKES 1 TREATMENT**

### Ingredients

1 nickel-sized dose of topical, full-spectrum, hemp-based CBD oil that has been tested for potency, purity, and quality

1 dose of magnesium chloride cream (the exact dose amount will depend on the brand you choose)

5 drops of lavender essential oil

### Method

1. Combine CBD, magnesium cream, and essential oil in your palm and rub hands together until they're fully mixed.
2. Apply to the back of the neck, side of the neck, jaw, shoulders, and upper back, giving yourself a little massage as you do.

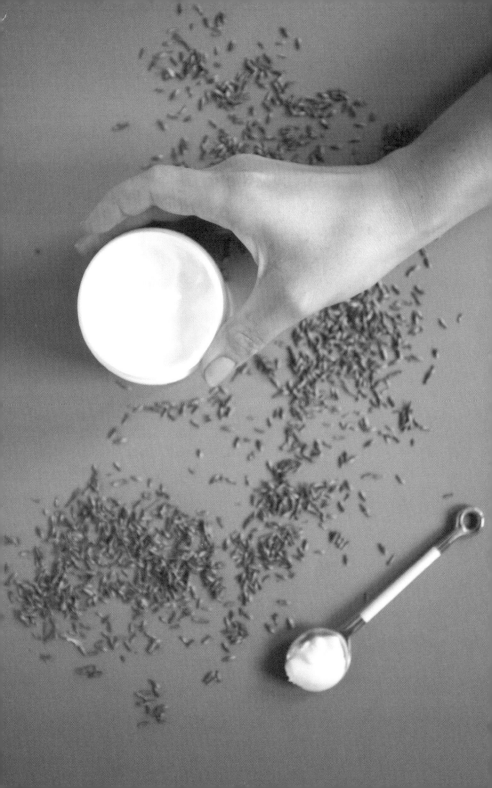

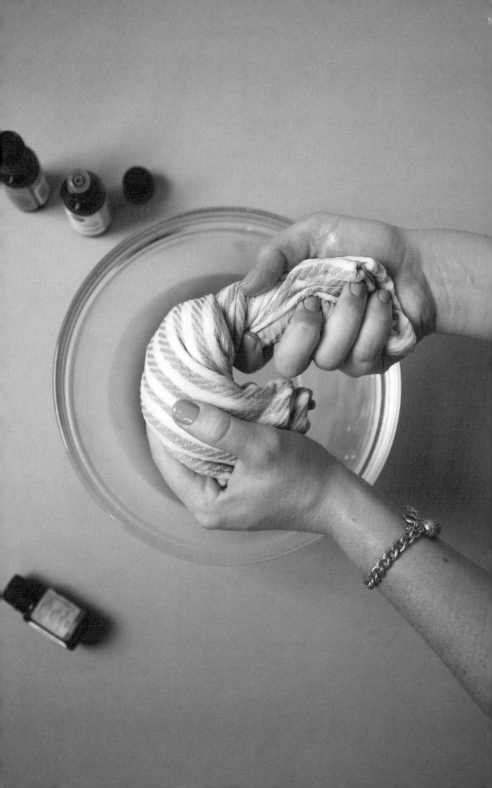

# Peppermint Headache Soak

*This peppermint remedy works well for me when I feel a tension headache coming on. We already know magnesium is great for headaches, but did you know that peppermint essential oil is a popular alternative option as well? Mint has amazing cooling properties and "targets headache pathophysiology in multiple ways" according to a German research study. I keep one or two of these treatments in the fridge so they're always ready when I need them. Try this one in combination with oral magnesium supplementation. In that case, you'd take magnesium in capsule form, and then do this treatment while the magnesium gets to work.*

**MAKES 1 TREATMENT**

### Ingredients

400 to 500 mg of magnesium in
    supplement capsule form

2 cups cold water

2 drops peppermint essential oil

1 clean washcloth

### Method

1. Take the oral magnesium supplement with a large cup of cold water.
2. Fill a large bowl with cool water, add essential oil, and stir. Dip a washcloth in the water and make sure it's fully soaked. Squeeze out excess water.
3. Lie down with the cool towel on your forehead or wherever your headache is located (avoiding the eyes, which can get irritated by the peppermint). I recommend resting with your eyes closed for 15 minutes and focusing on your breathing. This will help ease your tension and also allow time for the oral magnesium to start kicking in.
4. If you like to think ahead and want to place washcloths in the fridge so they're ready to go, triple this recipe, roll them up, and keep them in an airtight container.

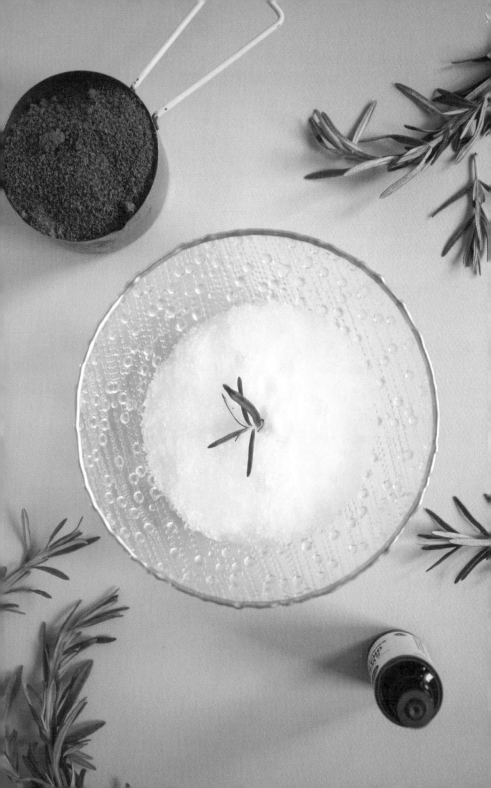

# Rosemary Orange Body Scrub

*Who doesn't love a good body scrub? Well, little did you know you can use magnesium sulfate salts as a base for your body scrub—saving you money and giving you the benefits of magnesium at the same time. This one is meant to be invigorating, and can be a great way to start your day. Rosemary is often used to improve focus (research has actually suggested it can improve memory and cognition), and orange smells, well, amazing.*

**MAKES 2 TREATMENTS**

## Ingredients

1 cup Epsom salts

1 cup brown sugar

½ cup coconut oil

5 drops sweet orange essential oil

1 or 2 sprigs of fresh rosemary

## Method

1. Combine Epsom salts and brown sugar in a large bowl. Add coconut oil and mix until fully incorporated.
2. Add orange essence and rosemary.
3. Transfer to a mason jar or other airtight container and allow a few hours for the rosemary to infuse the scrub. Keep the jar in your shower and don't forget to scrub your hands! They will feel like silk.

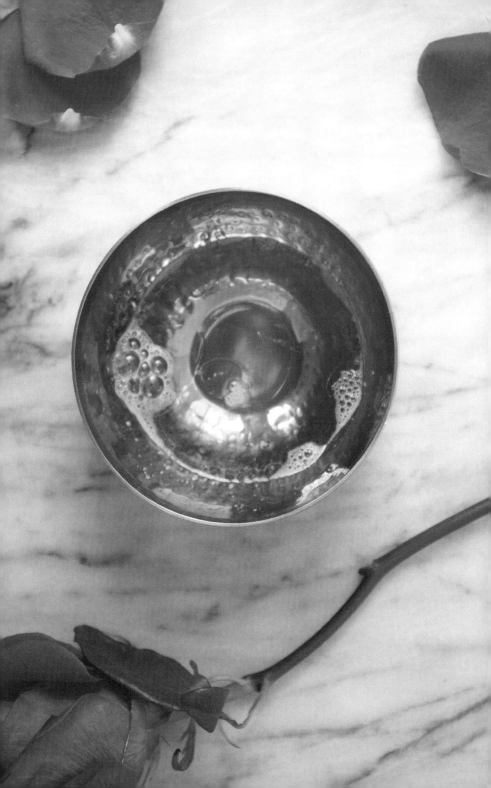

# Rose Oil Body Wash

*One of my fantastical life goals is for everything on and around me to effortlessly smell like roses. My perfume has rose hints, I diffuse rose oil in my apartment, buy fresh roses to just keep around, and have a very hard time not purchasing every beauty product that has the word rose (or even a picture of a rose) on it. I love this recipe because it lets me fully entertain my obsession. This rose oil body wash is perfect for the evenings. Every time I use it I get in bed feeling like a well-moisturized, relaxed (thank you, magnesium) baby who just happens to smell like a rose garden.*

**MAKES 1 TREATMENT**

### Ingredients

5 drops rose essential oil

1 dose magnesium chloride oil (the exact dose amount will depend on the brand you choose)

¼ cup apricot oil

¼ cup castile soap

### Method

1. Add all ingredients to a small mixing bowl and bring with you to the shower. Apply it just like normal body wash and rinse off with warm water. This one will leave you feeling extra hydrated because of the apricot oil, so there's probably no need to moisturize after.

# Tea Tree Oil Scalp Scrub

*I'm on a never-ending mission to make my hair bigger and more volu-minous. And that means I experiment with quite a few products and try to wash my hair only a few times a week (or less!). This also means that when I do wash my hair, I want it to feel* really *clean. I'd heard that magnesium sulfate can be good for removing residue from the hair, but I didn't really believe it until I tried it. This scrub has tea tree oil (a natural antimicrobial) and sweet almond oil. Take your time with this one, you deserve a nice scalp massage as much as the next person.*

**MAKES 1 TREATMENT**

### Ingredients

½ cup Epsom salts

3 to 5 drops tea tree oil

¼ cup sweet almond oil

### Method

1. Combine all ingredients in a small mixing bowl.
2. After you shampoo, apply scrub to head and massage into scalp gently, and then more vigorously.
3. Rinse thoroughly. If you're having trouble getting all the residue out, you can shampoo and rinse again.

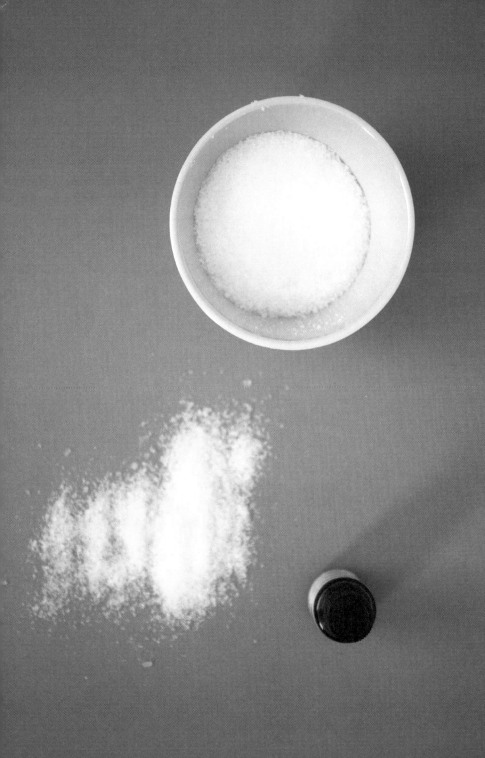

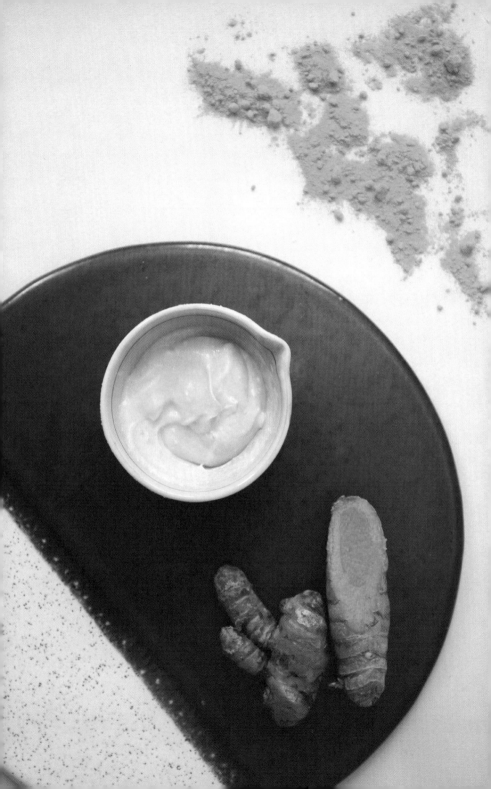

# Sore Muscle Balm

*Despite the lack of research backing up the benefits of arnica, it's one of my favorite natural remedies. It smells amazing, and I find that it's really helpful for bruises and muscle pain. Adding turmeric and frankincense essential oils can bring some helpful anti-inflammatory and pain-relieving properties to the mix. I like using this after a hard workout, or bringing it with me on vacation to use after all that walking! You can adjust the amount you use depending on how large of an area you want to cover. When using this balm, make sure you avoid your eyes and other sensitive areas. Also keep in mind that turmeric essential oil can leave a stain on the skin, although it will come out after a couple of washes.*

**MAKES 1 TREATMENT (perfect for an area the size of your feet and ankles or lower back)**

## Ingredients

1 dose magnesium cream (the exact dose amount will depend on the brand you choose)

1 teaspoon arnica gel or cream

3 drops turmeric essential oil

1 drop Frankincense essential oil

## Method

1. Combine magnesium cream with arnica cream in a small mixing bowl; add essential oils and stir.
2. Massage into the skin on the affected area, making sure to do it long enough that the cream fully absorbs.

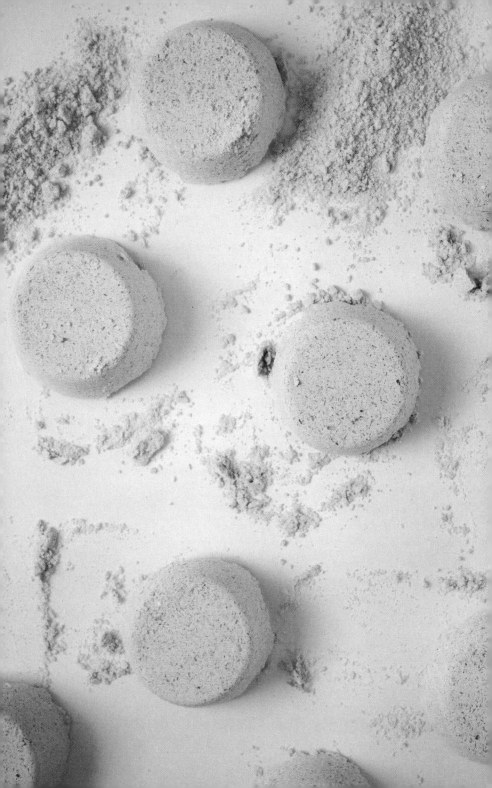

# Matcha Bath Bombs

*Matcha is basically supercharged green tea. It's made from pulverized green tea leaves, which contain added health benefits (as you're actually eating the leaf and not just drinking water infused with some of its properties). Unfortunately, matcha often makes me feel over-caffeinated, so I have to find other ways to take advantage of its antioxidant properties. A bath bomb is a good way to get some magnesium and matcha in my life without the racing heart. Keep in mind that while bath bombs are fun, they don't contain enough Epsom salts, so I add some extra to the bath itself when I'm looking to increase the effectiveness of the bomb.*

**MAKES MULTIPLE BOMBS**

### Ingredients

1 cup baking soda

½ cup citric acid

½ cup Epsom salts

½ cup cornstarch

1 tablespoon coconut oil, melted

1 teaspoon filtered water (don't use more than this or you'll activate the baking soda)

1 teaspoon matcha powder

### Method

1. Place baking soda, citric acid, Epsom salts, and cornstarch in a large bowl and mix until well combined.
2. In a small bowl, combine coconut oil and water.
3. Slowly pour the wet ingredients into the big bowl with the dry ingredients and mix thoroughly and evenly with your hands. This part is sometimes easier if you're wearing gloves. The mixture should resemble crumbly sand and should not feel wet to the touch. Once you reach this texture, add the matcha and mix.
4. Press the mixture firmly into greased molds (you can use bath bomb molds or any muffin pan) and let sit 24 to 48 hours. Once fully dry and hardened, carefully remove bath bombs from the mold. To use a bath bomb, just drop it directly into your bathtub while it's filling up. Store in an airtight container.

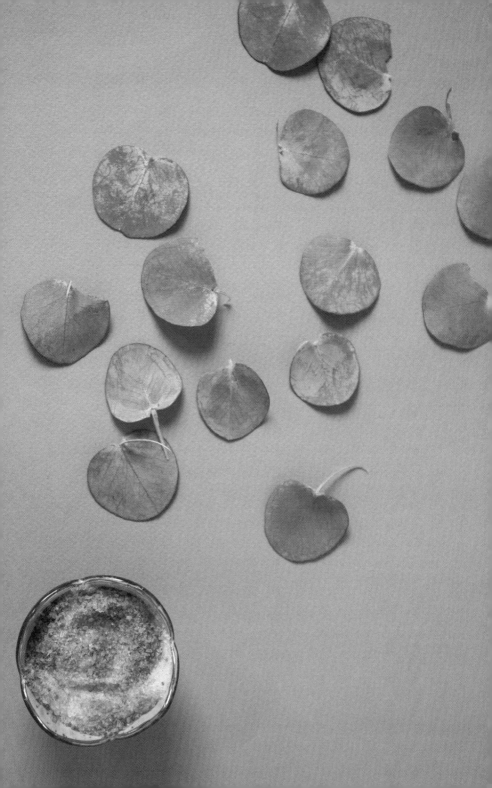

# Under-the-Weather Bath

*I love Manuka honey! This is my go-to if I'm feeling sniffle-y or my throat is getting a little bit scratchy. Eucalyptus is famous for its sinus-clearing abilities, and manuka honey has really strong anti-inflammatory and antimicrobial properties, which means it can help fight off certain viruses or bacteria. I like to lounge in this bath for at least 30 minutes and deeply inhale the eucalyptus scent. I love to add a few fresh eucalyptus leaves to the bath when I'm feeling fancy, they're even more fun than rose petals in my opinion.*

**MAKES 1 BATH**

### Ingredients

1 to 2 cups of Epsom salts (I like using Dr. Teal's Pure Epsom Salt Activated Charcoal for this recipe)

5 drops eucalyptus essential oil

1 tablespoon carrier oil (such as jojoba oil or coconut oil)

### Method

1. Run a warm bath and add Epsom salts while the faucet is still running; this will help them dissolve.
2. Add essential oil and carrier oil.
3. Swish water around with your hand until ingredients are fully incorporated and salts are totally dissolved.
4. Soak at least 20 to 30 minutes.

# Detox Bath

*There are some days when I just feel the need to cleanse. It might be that I just got home from vacation, I'm going through a stressful period at work, or it's the winter and I'm not getting to the gym as much as I'd like. Whatever the reason, I often turn to Aztec clay and apple cider vinegar. Both of these ingredients are famous for their detoxifying properties.*

**MAKES 1 BATH**

### Ingredients

1 to 2 cups of Epsom salts or magnesium chloride flakes

¼ cup Aztec clay

½ cup apple cider vinegar

5 drops lemon essential oil

1 tablespoon carrier oil (such as jojoba oil or coconut oil)

### Method

1. Run a warm bath and add Epsom salts while the faucet is still running; this will help them dissolve.
2. Add clay, vinegar, and essential oil in carrier oil. Mix with your hand or a large wooden spoon until fully incorporated.
3. Swish water around with your hand until ingredients are fully incorporated and salts are totally dissolved.
4. Soak for 20 to 30 minutes.

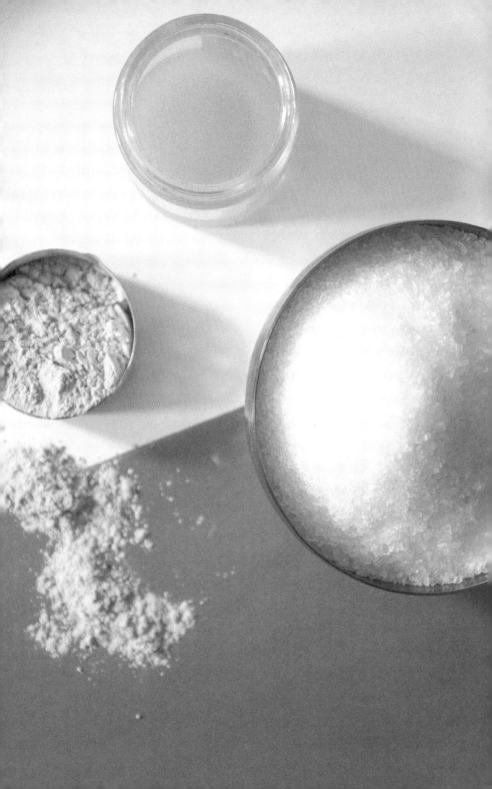

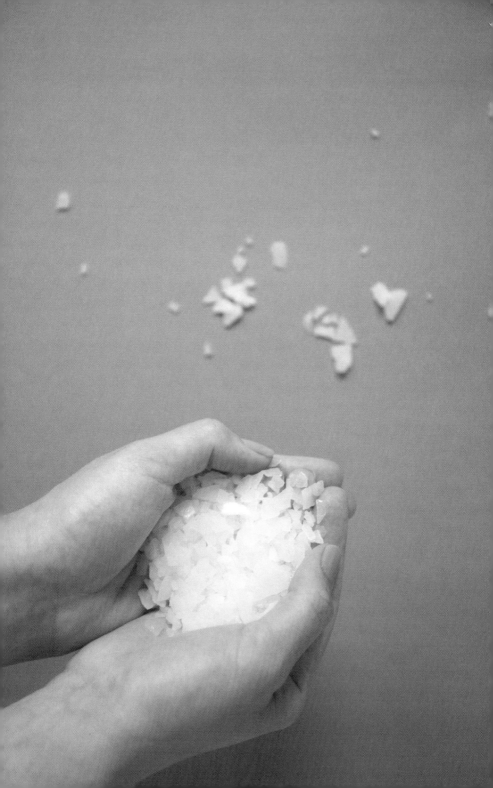

# Post-Workout Bath

*If an electrolyte drink isn't your thing, this post-workout bath might be for you. I use it in the evening after a tough workout or to help relieve my tiredness the next day. If you're feeling really brave, dissolve the magnesium salt and sea salt in a little bit of hot water at the bottom of the tub, and then fill the rest up with cold water and ice. It won't be quite as relaxing as some of the other baths, but it'll get the job done.*

**MAKES 1 BATH**

### Ingredients

1 to 2 cups magnesium salt (I like using Ancient Minerals Magnesium Bath Flakes)

5 drops lemongrass essential oil

1 tablespoon carrier oil (such as jojoba oil or coconut oi)

¼ cup Himalayan pink sea salt

### Method

1. Run a warm bath and add salts while the faucet is still running; this will help them dissolve.
2. Add lemongrass essential oil and sea salt.
3. Swish water around with your hand until ingredients are fully incorporated and salts are totally dissolved.
4. Soak 20 to 30 minutes.
5. For the ice bath, add hot water to the bottom of the bathtub and dissolve salts, then fill the rest with cold water and add ice as needed. Soak for no more than 6 to 8 minutes.

# Skin-Soothing Bath

*Whether it be from a particularly dry winter, an allergic reaction, a sunburn, or a chronic issue, sometimes our skin is just unhappy. This bath is for those days. It's formulated with only the most calming ingredients such as anti-inflammatory and skin-soothing manuka honey, antioxidant-rich vitamin E oil, and nourishing oatmeal. This bath helps me get through New York City winters, and I'm forever grateful for it.*

**MAKES 1 BATH**

### Ingredients

1 cup oats, dry and unflavored

1 to 2 cups Epsom salts or magnesium chloride flakes

1 tablespoon manuka honey

1 dose vitamin E oil (the exact dose amount will depend on the brand you choose)

### Method

1. Pour oats into a blender and blend until they're ground to a fine powder.
2. Run a warm bath and add Epsom salts while the faucet is still running; this will help them dissolve.
3. Add oat powder, manuka honey, and vitamin E oil. Swish water around with your hand or large wooden spoon until ingredients are fully incorporated and salts are totally dissolved.
4. Soak 20 to 30 minutes.

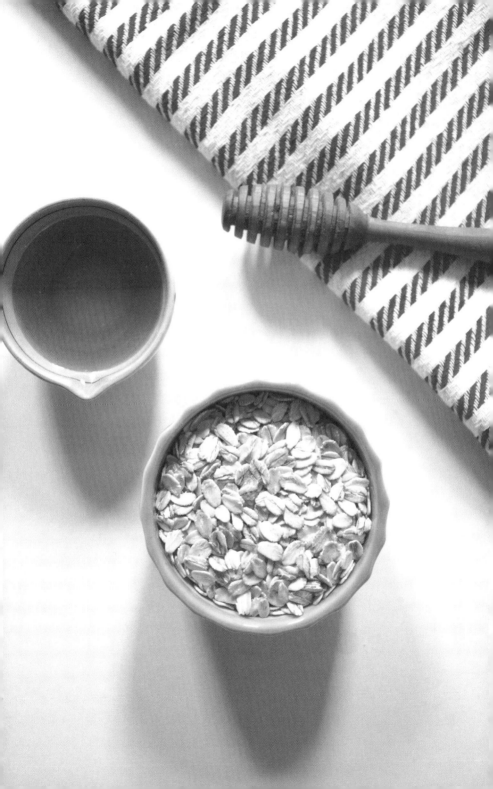

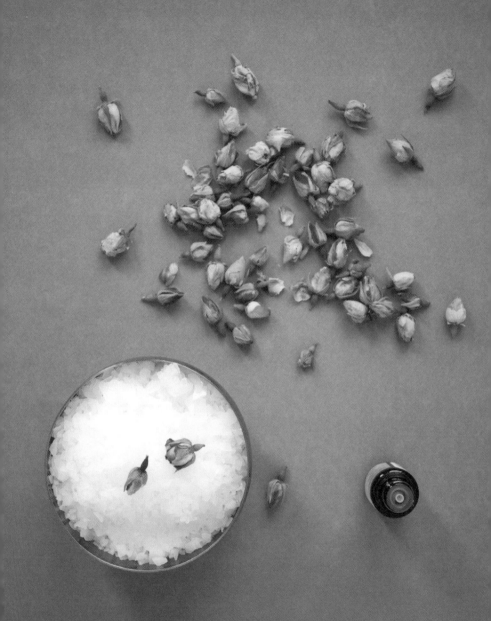

# Hormone-Balancing Bath

*It's that time of the month and nothing sounds better than a hot bath to get some relief from bloating, cramps, and general discomfort. Cue this hormone-balancing bath. You can take this bath any time of the month, but it is especially welcome at this particular moment. Clary sage is famous for hormone balance, and chamomile can help soothe your body and promote relaxation. Make sure to add the full dose of Epsom salts in this one so you can get the full benefits.*

**MAKES 1 BATH**

### Ingredients

1 to 2 cups Epsom salts or magnesium chloride flakes

5 drops chamomile essential oil

3 drops clary sage essential oil

1 tablespoon carrier oil (such as jojoba oil or coconut oil)

1 tablespoon coconut milk powder

### Method

1. Run a warm bath and add Epsom salts while the faucet is still running; this will help them dissolve.
2. Add chamomile and clary sage essential oils along with carrier oil and coconut milk powder.
3. Swish water around with your hand until ingredients are fully incorporated and salts are totally dissolved.
4. Soak 20 to 30 minutes.

# Libido-Boosting Bubble Bath

*Ready for a little romance? We could all probably use a little more of it in our lives. Cue this bath recipe, which can be enjoyed solo or with a partner. Epsom salts are a great way to wind down, and ylang ylang is often recommended by essential oil experts to boost libido. The roses add a little bit of luxury to this already-sweet-smelling bath. Bonus: The sweet almond oil will leave your skin hydrated and silky smooth. Need I say more?*

**MAKES 1 BATH**

### Ingredients

1 to 2 cups Epsom salts or magnesium chloride flakes

3 drops ylang ylang essential oil

1 tablespoon carrier oil (I like using sweet almond oil)

2 cups rose petals (optional)

### Method

1. Run a warm bath and add Epsom salts while the faucet is still running; this will help them dissolve.
2. Add essential oil and carrier oil.
3. Swish water around with your hand until ingredients are fully incorporated and salts are totally dissolved. Add rose petals, if using.
4. Soak 20 to 30 minutes.

# CONCLUSION
## Some Final Thoughts on Magnesium

So there you have it! If you've gotten this far, I hope you feel that you've learned more about magnesium. Actually, scratch that: I hope you feel like you've learned more about the epidemic of chronic stress, the history of spiritual bathing, the science of electrolytes, the ins and outs of calcium-magnesium balance, the side effects of common over-the-counter remedies, *and* magnesium—and that's just a few of the many topics we covered all at once. Thanks for sticking with me!

As you were reading this book, you may have been surprised by some of the things you learned about our medical system and the way we approach health care in the United States. This book might have forced you to ask some questions about our conventional health care system and the type of care you've been getting. That's a good thing! If you bought this book, I think it's safe to assume that you're an empowered individual who wants to play an active role in your own health—and knowledge is power.

When it comes down to it, the responsibility falls on us to make sure we're living our healthiest lives. This means a few different things: We can't just assume that the food that is available to us is healthy (it's probably not). We can't assume that we'll get any exercise at all if we don't consciously plan for it and make it happen (thanks to sedentary living, long work hours in front of the computer, and our driving culture). We can't assume that our doctor is aware of lifestyle changes—such as dietary changes, supplements, herbs, or other alternative remedies—that might help with our condition. And we can't *assume* they'll think to suggest supplementing with magnesium for the conditions described in Chapter 4. This doesn't mean we can't trust anyone with medical advice, nor does it mean we have to resort to growing all our food in our own backyard. Rather, taking personal responsibility for our health just means we have to be active players in our own wellness and to pay attention to what's going on.

Admittedly, it can be overwhelming and anxiety-provoking to be in charge of it all. Why does it have to fall on us to make sure we're getting the best health care possible? Aren't we already suffering enough when we're not feeling our best? I hear you. The shortcomings of both conventional and alternative medicine can be frustrating. And I mean *really frustrating*. This is especially true when you learn that the people suffering the most from the current system are the patients and the doctors. Most doctors are sleep deprived, unbelievably stressed, rushed with every patient, and restricted by pharmaceutical companies and insurance companies—which both have a lot of influence over patient care—and who knows how many *hundreds of thousands* of dollars of student loan debt. Doctors have some of the highest suicide rates of any profession, and many of them are frustrated by the lack of education about lifestyle changes and nutrition that they received in medical school. In short, we can't go blaming doctors for our health care woes, because many of them would like to see many of the same changes we want.

This brings me to the final takeaway of this book, which is interestingly not about reducing stress, prioritizing self-care, or even taking magnesium. Instead, I'd like to leave you with a little bit of savviness so that you can *always* ask questions about your health. What are these questions? Just a few examples: "Are there any dietary changes I could make that would improve my condition?" and "What role might stress play in how well I'm feeling?" and "Can I find a doctor who really listens to me and is willing to think outside the box?" The questions might seem simple, but asking them can set you on the path to wellness and can make the difference between years of suffering and not.

So keep asking your doctor about nutrition and lifestyle change; let them know it's important to you to exhaust all natural or lifestyle changes before taking a pill—and let them know that you're motivated enough to make the necessary changes and stick to them (if you are, of course). Keep letting them know what natural remedies you're trying and, of course, which supplements you're taking. Ask them about magnesium and make sure they hear you.

At the same time, when you go to your alternative medicine practitioners ask them about the science of what they're doing, whether it be acupuncture, Reiki, naturopathy, and so forth. Ask them about safety concerns and the research that supports the modality or technique. Ask them if they've ever teamed up with a conventional medicine doctor to better treat patients, or if they're affiliated with any hospitals or take insurance. I believe that the space between conventional and alternative medicine is where truly great health care lives, and that bridging the gap between the two—pulling on the knowledge and valuable resources both can provide—is the quickest way to improve health care for everyone. And at the end of the day, can't we all agree that that's the ultimate goal?

# RESOURCES

Abbasi, Behnood, Masud Kimiagar, Khosro Sadeghniiat, Minoo M. Shirazi, Mehdi Hedayati, and Bahram Rashidkhani. "The Effect of Magnesium Supplementation on Primary Insomnia in Elderly: A Double-Blind Placebo-Controlled Clinical Trial." *Journal of Research in Medical Sciences: The Official Journal of Isfahan University of Medical Sciences* 17, no. 12 (December 2012): 1161–69.

Andermann, G., and M. Dietz. "The Bioavailability and Pharmacokinetics of Three Zinc Salts: Zinc Pantothenate, Zinc Sulfate and Zinc Orotate." *European Journal of Drug Metabolism and Pharmacokinetics* 7, no. 3 (1982): 233–39.

Arranz, Laura-Isabel, Miguel-Ángel Canela, and Magda Rafecas. "Dietary Aspects in Fibromyalgia Patients: Results of a Survey on Food Awareness, Allergies, and Nutritional Supplementation." *Rheumatology International* 32, no. 9 (September 2012): 2615–21. https://doi.org/10.1007/s00296-011-2010-z.

Aydin, Hasan, Oğuzhan Deyneli, Dilek Yavuz, Hülya Gözü, Nilgün Mutlu, Işik Kaygusuz, and Sema Akalin. "Short-Term Oral Magnesium Supplementation Suppresses Bone Turnover in Postmenopausal Osteoporotic Women." *Biological Trace Element Research* 133, no. 2 (February 2010): 136–43. https://doi.org/10.1007/s12011-009-8416-8.

Bagis, Selda, Mehmet Karabiber, Ismet As, Lülüfer Tamer, Canan Erdogan, and Ayçe Atalay. "Is Magnesium Citrate Treatment Effective on Pain, Clinical Parameters and Functional Status in Patients with Fibromyalgia?" *Rheuma-*

*tology International* 33, no. 1 (January 2013): 167–72. https://doi.org/10.1007/s00296-011-2334-8.

Barbagallo, M., and L. J. Dominguez. "Magnesium and Aging." *Current Pharmaceutical Design* 16, no. 7 (2010): 832–39.

Belluci, Marina Montosa, Gabriela Giro, Ricardo Andrés Landazuri Del Barrio, Rosa Maria Rodrigues Pereira, Elcio Marcantonio, and Silvana Regina Perez Orrico. "Effects of Magnesium Intake Deficiency on Bone Metabolism and Bone Tissue around Osseointegrated Implants." *Clinical Oral Implants Research* 22, no. 7 (July 2011): 716–21. https://doi.org/10.1111/j.1600-0501.2010.02046.x.

Bergman, E. A., L. K. Massey, K. J. Wise, and D. J. Sherrard. "Effects of Dietary Caffeine on Renal Handling of Minerals in Adult Women." *Life Sciences* 47, no. 6 (1990): 557–64.

Bertakis, K. D., R. Azari, L. J. Helms, E. J. Callahan, and J. A. Robbins. "Gender Differences in the Utilization of Health Care Services." *The Journal of Family Practice* 49, no. 2 (February 2000): 147–52.

Bolland, Mark J., William Leung, Vicky Tai, Sonja Bastin, Greg D. Gamble, Andrew Grey, and Ian R. Reid. "Calcium Intake and Risk of Fracture: Systematic Review." *BMJ* 351 (September 29, 2015): h4580. https://doi.org/10.1136/bmj.h4580.

Boskey, A. L., C. M. Rimnac, M. Bansal, M. Federman, J. Lian, and B. D. Boyan. "Effect of Short-Term Hypomagnesemia on the Chemical and Mechanical Properties of Rat Bone." *Journal of Orthopaedic Research: Official Publication of the Orthopaedic Research Society* 10, no. 6 (November 1992): 774–83. https://doi.org/10.1002/jor.1100100605.

Castiglioni, Sara, and Jeanette A. M. Maier. "Magnesium and Cancer: A Dangerous Liaison." *Magnesium Research* 24, no. 3 (September 2011): S92–100. https://doi.org/10.1684/mrh.2011.0285.

Chen, Esther H., Frances S. Shofer, Anthony J. Dean, Judd E. Hollander, William G. Baxt, Jennifer L. Robey, Keara L. Sease, and Angela M. Mills. "Gender Disparity in Analgesic Treatment of Emergency Department Patients with Acute Abdominal Pain." *Academic Emergency Medicine* 15, no. 5 (May 1, 2008): 414–18. https://doi.org/10.1111/j.1553-2712.2008.00100.x.

Cox, I. M., M. J. Campbell, and D. Dowson. "Red Blood Cell Magnesium and Chronic Fatigue Syndrome." *The Lancet* 337, no. 8744 (March 30, 1991): 757–60. https://doi.org/10.1016/0140-6736(91)91371-Z.

Dai, Qi, Xiao-Ou Shu, Xinqing Deng, Yong-Bing Xiang, Honglan Li, Gong Yang, Martha J. Shrubsole, et al. "Modifying Effect of Calcium/Magnesium Intake Ratio and Mortality: A Population-Based Cohort Study." *BMJ Open* 3, no. 2 (January 1, 2013): e002111. https://doi.org/10.1136/bmjopen-2012-002111.

Dupont, Christophe, Alain Campagne, and Florence Constant. "Efficacy and Safety of a Magnesium Sulfate-Rich Natural Mineral Water for Patients with Functional Constipation." *Clinical Gastroenterology and Hepatology: The Official Clinical Practice Journal of the American Gastroenterological Association* 12, no. 8 (August 2014): 1280–87. https://doi.org/10.1016/j.cgh.2013.12.005.

Elin, Ronald J. "Assessment of Magnesium Status for Diagnosis and Therapy." *Magnesium Research* 23, no. 4 (December 2010): S194–98. https://doi.org/10.1684/mrh.2010.0213.

Erlich, Jeffrey C., Bingni W. Brunton, Chunyu A. Duan, Timothy D. Hanks, and Carlos D. Brody. "Distinct Effects of Prefrontal and Parietal Cortex Inactivations on an Accumulation of Evidence Task in the Rat." *eLife* 4. https://doi.org/10.7554/eLife.05457 (accessed September 17, 2018).

Facchinetti, F., G. Sances, P. Borella, A. R. Genazzani, and G. Nappi. "Magnesium Prophylaxis of Menstrual Migraine: Effects on Intracellular Magnesium." *Headache* 31, no. 5 (May 1991): 298–301.

Fan, Ming-Sheng, Fang-Jie Zhao, Susan J. Fairweather-Tait, Paul R. Poulton, Sarah J. Dunham, and Steve P. McGrath. "Evidence of Decreasing Mineral Density in Wheat Grain over the Last 160 Years." *Journal of Trace Elements in Medicine and Biology: Organ of the Society for Minerals and Trace Elements (GMS)* 22, no. 4 (2008): 315–24. https://doi.org/10.1016/j.jtemb.2008.07.002.

Gallagher, R. Michael, and Robert Kunkel. "Migraine Medication Attributes Important for Patient Compliance: Concerns About Side Effects May Delay Treatment." *Headache: The Journal of Head and Face Pain* 43, no. 1 (2003): 36–43. https://doi.org/10.1046/j.1526-4610.2003.03006.x.

Griffin, Annaliese. "Women Are Flocking to Wellness Because Modern Medicine Still Doesn't Take Them Seriously." *Quartz.* https://qz.com/1006387/women-are-flocking-to-wellness-because-traditional-medicine-still-doesnt-take-them-seriously/ (accessed September 17, 2018).

Harvard T. H. Chan, Harvard School of Public Health. "Doctors Need More Nutrition Education." News, May 9, 2017. www.hsph.harvard.edu/news/hsph-in-the-news/doctors-nutrition-education/ (accessed May 9, 2017).

He, Ka, Kiang Liu, Martha L. Daviglus, Steven J. Morris, Catherine M. Loria, Linda Van Horn, David R. Jacobs, and Peter J. Savage. "Magnesium Intake and Incidence of Metabolic Syndrome among Young Adults." *Circulation* 113, no. 13 (April 4, 2006): 1675–82. https://doi.org/10.1161/CIRCULATIONAHA.105.588327.

Hornyak, M., U. Voderholzer, F. Hohagen, M. Berger, and D. Riemann. "Magnesium Therapy for Periodic Leg Movements-Related Insomnia and Restless Legs Syndrome: An Open Pilot Study." *Sleep* 21, no. 5 (August 1, 1998): 501–5.

Jahnen-Dechent, Wilhelm, and Markus Ketteler. "Magnesium Basics." *Clinical Kidney Journal* 5, no. Suppl 1 (February 2012): i3–14. https://doi.org/10.1093/ndtplus/sfr163.

Johns Hopkins Medicine. "Calcium Supplements May Damage the Heart." October 11, 2016. www.hopkinsmedicine.org/news/media/releases/calcium_supplements_may_damage_the_heart. (accessed September 17, 2018).

Johnson, S. "The Multifaceted and Widespread Pathology of Magnesium Deficiency." *Medical Hypotheses* 56, no. 2 (February 1, 2001): 163–70. https://doi.org/10.1054/mehy.2000.1133.

Kozielec, T., and B. Starobrat-Hermelin. "Assessment of Magnesium Levels in

Children with Attention Deficit Hyperactivity Disorder (ADHD)." *Magnesium Research* 10, no. 2 (June 1997): 143–48.

Kutsal, Ebru, Cumhur Aydemir, Nilufer Eldes, Fatma Demirel, Recep Polat, Ozan Taspnar, and Eyup Kulah. "Severe Hypermagnesemia as a Result of Excessive Cathartic Ingestion in a Child Without Renal Failure." *Pediatric Emergency Care* 23, no. 8 (August 2007): 570–72. https://doi.org/10.1097/PEC.0b013e31812eef1c.

Laconi, E., A. Denda, P. M. Rao, S. Rajalakshmi, P. Pani, and D. S. Sarma. "Studies on Liver Tumor Promotion in the Rat by Orotic Acid: Dose and Minimum Exposure Time Required for Dietary Orotic Acid to Promote Hepatocarcinogenesis." *Carcinogenesis* 14, no. 9 (September 1993): 1771–75.

Larsson, Susanna C., Nicola Orsini, and Alicja Wolk. "Dietary Magnesium Intake and Risk of Stroke: A Meta-Analysis of Prospective Studies." *The American Journal of Clinical Nutrition* 95, no. 2 (February 2012): 362–66. https://doi.org/10.3945/ajcn.111.022376.

Levav, A. L., L. Chan, and R. J. Wapner. "Long-Term Magnesium Sulfate Tocolysis and Maternal Osteoporosis in a Triplet Pregnancy: A Case Report." *American Journal of Perinatology* 15, no. 1 (January 1998): 43–46. https://doi.org/10.1055/s-2007-993897.

Liu, Katherine A., and Natalie A. Dipietro Mager. "Women's Involvement in Clinical Trials: Historical Perspective and Future Implications." *Pharmacy Practice* 14, no. 1 (2016). https://doi.org/10.18549/PharmPract.2016.01.708.

Mazur, Andrzej, Jeanette A. M. Maier, Edmond Rock, Elyett Gueux, Wojciech Nowacki, and Yves Rayssiguier. "Magnesium and the Inflammatory Response: Potential Physiopathological Implications." *Archives of Biochemistry and Biophysics* 458, no. 1 (February 1, 2007): 48–56. https://doi.org/10.1016/j.abb.2006.03.031.

McGuire, J. K., M. S. Kulkarni, and H. P. Baden. "Fatal Hypermagnesemia in a Child Treated with Megavitamin/Megamineral Therapy." *Pediatrics* 105, no. 2 (February 2000): E18.

National Institutes of Health, Office of Dietary Supplements. "Magnesium: Fact Sheet for Health Professionals." https://ods.od.nih.gov/factsheets/Magnesium-HealthProfessional (accessed September 17, 2018).

Nerbrand, Christina, Lars Agréus, Ragnhild Arvidsson Lenner, Per Nyberg, and Kurt Svärdsudd. "The Influence of Calcium and Magnesium in Drinking Water and Diet on Cardiovascular Risk Factors in Individuals Living in Hard and Soft Water Areas with Differences in Cardiovascular Mortality." *BMC Public Health* 3 (June 18, 2003): 21. https://doi.org/10.1186/1471-2458-3-21.

Nielsen, Forrest H. "Effects of Magnesium Depletion on Inflammation in Chronic Disease." *Current Opinion in Clinical Nutrition and Metabolic Care* 17, no. 6 (November 2014): 525–30. https://doi.org/10.1097/MCO.0000000000000093.

Otberg, Nina, Heike Richter, Hans Schaefer, Ulrike Blume-Peytavi, Wolfram Sterry, and Jürgen Lademann. "Variations of Hair Follicle Size and Distribution in Different Body Sites." *The Journal of Investigative Dermatology* 122, no. 1 (January 2004): 14–19. https://doi.org/10.1046/j.0022-202X.2003.22110.x.

Piccolo, Jennifer, and Jill M. Kolesar. "Prevention and Treatment of Chemotherapy-Induced Peripheral Neuropathy." *American Journal of Health-System Pharmacy: AJHP: Official Journal of the American Society of Health-System Pharmacists* 71, no. 1 (January 1, 2014): 19–25. https://doi.org/10.2146/ajhp130126.

Piovesan, Damiano, Giuseppe Profiti, Pier Luigi Martelli, and Rita Casadio. "The Human 'Magnesome': Detecting Magnesium Binding Sites on Human Proteins." *BMC Bioinformatics* 13, no. Suppl 14 (September 7, 2012): S10. https://doi.org/10.1186/1471-2105-13-S14-S10.

Popoviciu, L., B. Aşgian, D. Delast-Popoviciu, A. Alexandrescu, S. Petruţiu, and I. Bagathal. "Clinical, EEG, Electromyographic and Polysomnographic Studies in Restless Legs Syndrome Caused by Magnesium Deficiency." *Romanian Journal of Neurology and Psychiatry* (*Revue Roumaine De Neurologie Et Psychiatrie*) 31, no. 1 (March 1993): 55–61.

Reynolds, Margaret. "Stress in Health and Disease." *The Yale Journal of Biology and Medicine* 81, no. 1 (March 2008): 53–54.

Rondón, L. J., A. M. Privat, L. Daulhac, N. Davin, A. Mazur, J. Fialip, A. Eschalier, and C. Courteix. "Magnesium Attenuates Chronic Hypersensitivity and Spinal Cord NMDA Receptor Phosphorylation in a Rat Model of Diabetic Neuropathic Pain." *The Journal of Physiology* 588, no. 21 (November 1, 2010): 4205–15. https://doi.org/10.1113/jphysiol.2010.197004.

Rude, Robert K., Frederick R. Singer, and Helen E. Gruber. "Skeletal and Hormonal Effects of Magnesium Deficiency." *Journal of the American College of Nutrition* 28, no. 2 (April 2009): 131–41.

Schuette, S. A., B. A. Lashner, and M. Janghorbani. "Bioavailability of Magnesium Diglycinate vs Magnesium Oxide in Patients with Ileal Resection." *JPEN. Journal of Parenteral and Enteral Nutrition* 18, no. 5 (October 1994): 430–35. https://doi.org/10.1177/0148607194018005430.

Sills, Sheila, Christine Roffe, Peter Crome, and Peter Jones. "Randomised, Cross-Over, Placebo Controlled Trial of Magnesium Citrate in the Treatment of Chronic Persistent Leg Cramps." *Medical Science Monitor* 8, no. 5 (May 15, 2002): CR326–30.

Simental-Mendía, Luis E., Martha Rodríguez-Morán, and Fernando Guerrero-Romero. "Oral Magnesium Supplementation Decreases C-Reactive Protein Levels in Subjects with Prediabetes and Hypomagnesemia: A Clinical Randomized Double-Blind Placebo-Controlled Trial." *Archives of Medical Research* 45, no. 4 (May 2014): 325–30. https://doi.org/10.1016/j.arcmed.2014.04.006.

Stepura, O. B., and A. I. Martynow. "Magnesium Orotate in Severe Congestive Heart Failure (MACH)." *International Journal of Cardiology* 134, no. 1 (May 1, 2009): 145–47.

Sun-Edelstein, Christina, and Alexander Mauskop. "Role of Magnesium in the Pathogenesis and Treatment of Migraine." *Expert Review of Neurotherapeutics* 9, no. 3 (March 2009): 369–79. https://doi.org/10.1586/14737175.9.3.369.

Tong, Garrison M., and Robert K. Rude. "Magnesium Deficiency in Critical Illness." *Journal of Intensive Care Medicine* 20, no. 1 (February 2005): 3–17. https://doi.org/10.1177/0885066604271539.

Walker, A. F., M. C. De Souza, M. F. Vickers, S. Abeyasekera, M. L. Collins, and L. A. Trinca. "Magnesium Supplementation Alleviates Premenstrual Symptoms of Fluid Retention." *Journal of Women's Health* 7, no. 9 (November 1998): 1157–65.

Wienecke, Elmar, and Claudia Nolden. "[Long-Term HRV Analysis Shows Stress Reduction by Magnesium Intake]." *MMW Fortschritte der Medizin* 158, no. Suppl 6 (December 2016): 12–16. https://doi.org/10.1007/s15006-016-9054-7.

Witkowski, Michał, Jane Hubert, and Andrzej Mazur. "Methods of Assessment of Magnesium Status in Humans: A Systematic Review." *Magnesium Research* 24, no. 4 (December 2011): 163–80. https://doi.org/10.1684/mrh.2011.0292.

Yamadera, Wataru, Kentaro Inagawa, Shintaro Chiba, Makoto Bannai, Michio Takahashi, and Kazuhiko Nakayama. "Glycine Ingestion Improves Subjective Sleep Quality in Human Volunteers, Correlating with Polysomnographic Changes." *Sleep and Biological Rhythms* 5, no. 2 (April 1, 2007): 126–31. https://doi.org/10.1111/j.1479-8425.2007.00262.x.

Zarean, Elaheh, and Amal Tarjan. "Effect of Magnesium Supplement on Pregnancy Outcomes: A Randomized Control Trial." *Advanced Biomedical Research* 6 (August 31, 2017). https://doi.org/10.4103/2277-9175.213879.

Zofková, I., and R. L. Kancheva. "The Relationship between Magnesium and Calciotropic Hormones." *Magnesium Research* 8, no. 1 (March 1995): 77–84.

# ACKNOWLEDGMENTS

Thank you to my parents, who continue to support me every single day in more ways than one. I wouldn't be anywhere if it wasn't for you!

Thank you so much to my agent, Anna; you have helped keep me sane and I'm so grateful!

Thank you to my editor, Róisín, for helping me write the best books possible and become an all-around better writer.

Thank you to Lucia for coming to New York City to lend her photography expertise. Somehow it ended up being the most fun part of this process. I don't like to imagine what life would be like if we hadn't been neighbors that first year in Buist!

Thank you to Liz Moody for the help with ideas, feedback, recipes, art direction, supplies, and emotional support. Basically everything. Thank you for being such a big part of my success.

Thank you to Hannah, Hannah M, Bobbitt, Zack, Elle, Emma, Ray, Lauren, Lindsay, Uncle Jim, and all my other friends and family members who have been so generous with their support and loving words.

Thank you to the editorial team at mbg for the support and love this year. You all are the best!

# INDEX